Wisconsin Publications in the
History of Science and Medicine
Number 6

General Editors

William Coleman
David C. Lindberg
Ronald L. Numbers

Yellow Fever in the North

The Methods of
Early Epidemiology

William Coleman

The University of Wisconsin Press

Published 1987

The University of Wisconsin Press
114 North Murray Street
Madison, Wisconsin 53715

The University of Wisconsin Press, Ltd.
1 Gower Street
London WC1E 6HA, England

First printing

Printed in the United States of America

For LC CIP information see the colophon

ISBN 0-299-11110-5 (cloth); 0-299-11114-8 (paper)

In Memory of My Mother
Ruth Elizabeth Morgan
and
For My Aunt
Esther Catharine Morgan

Contents

Illustrations

Acknowledgments

AS EVER, many persons and institutions have assisted me in the course of my work. I offer special thanks to Dorothy Whitcomb of the Middleton Medical Library, Madison, and Dorothy Hanks at the National Library of Medicine, Bethesda. I am no less indebted to helpful staff members at the Bibliothèque nationale, Paris; the Wellcome Institute of the History of Medicine, London; the medical division of the Universitätsbibliothek, Düsseldorf; the Staatsbibliothek Preussischer Kulturbesitz, Berlin; and, especially, the Library of the Zentrum für interdisziplinäre Forschung and the Universitätsbibliothek, Bielefeld. John Neu and Jean Théodoridès have offered their usual and greatly appreciated assistance, and I am particularly grateful to John M. Eyler and Wilbur G. Downs, who each read a draft of this work with a critical and helpful eye. Two referees devoted uncommon attention to my manuscript and they will find their mark throughout the ensuing book; my thanks to their anonymous selves. I appreciate, too, the assistance of the many persons who aided me in obtaining the illustrations. Lori Grant brought this book from pencil to typescript: I have no greater debt. Portions of chapters 4 and 5 have appeared in the *Bulletin of the History of Medicine* (58 [1984]: 145–163) and are published here in revised form with the kind permission of the editor and the Johns Hopkins University Press. Research support from the National Library of Medicine (Grant LM 03474) and a fellowship from the Stiftung Volkswagenwerk, Hanover, are gratefully acknowledged. Above all, I express my gratitude to the family of Carol Dickson, whose generous gift to the University of Wisconsin has greatly assisted my research.

Madison, Wisconsin
December 1986

Introduction

THE STUDY OF communicable disease in the twentieth century is closely associated with the germ theory of disease. Physicians and epidemiologists today emphasize the pathogenic effects of the causal agent of a disease, commonly a microorganism, and they explore how that agent moves through a human population. This approach provides an essential basis for epidemiological reasoning. It is an etiological basis and in this form is quite new, being the product of the medical revolution inaugurated by experimental bacteriology in the 1870s and 1880s.

Epidemiology, however, long antedates the germ theory of disease. With strong roots in classical Greek medicine, the science gained valuable experience in dealing with a host of epidemic diseases over long centuries of subsequent development. By the nineteenth century, epidemiology had attained early maturity, and the consideration of the etiology of disease remained among its many concerns. Some early epidemiologists had, in fact, entertained the idea of a microscopical, living cause of disease. This notion, however, was purely hypothetical; the existence and action of such an agent could in no case be demonstrated in an unequivocal manner. Probably the great majority of epidemiologists favored a different causal explanation, namely, disease travels through the community by means of a harmful atmospheric influence. This, the so-called miasmatic doctrine, assumed that the atmosphere, after receiving noxious substances arising from inorganic sources or from putrefying organic materials, conveys the poison to susceptible persons. When local conditions were suitable, such a miasma could induce a serious epidemic.

It is an untoward result of the triumph of the germ theory of disease that the development of epidemiology has come to be viewed primarily through the spectacles of that theory and of etiological reasoning in general. This is misleading, even false. Prior to 1880, etiological explanations for communicable disease were numerous and varied, but these theories were not easily reconciled with one another and they struggled, usually unsuccessfully, to remain both comprehensive and self-consistent. They also suffered severely from a dearth of relevant and reliable empirical evidence.

In the case of yellow fever, the nineteenth century favored a noncontagionist view of causation: transmission was effected not by person-to-person contact (contagion) but by the movement of a morbid influence (miasma) through the atmosphere. The precise source of this influence was often left unspecified. As the following discussion will reveal, even those who despaired of solving the causal question were compelled to take a stand on these issues. It deserves special note, however, that this was not their, or the epidemiologist's, primary concern. To these inquirers, the foremost need was to trace the movement of an epidemic disease and to determine from the information thus gained the characteristic epidemic behavior of the disease. Then, making use of their discoveries, they sought to find appropriate and economical means to halt the spread of the disease and to prevent future epidemics.

On the eve of the germ theory of disease, in 1861 and 1865, two physicians — today little known but each in his lifetime a figure of high reputation — examined two yellow-fever epidemics in unexpected locations. Unsurprisingly, neither could resolve the etiological question and each remained loyal to the noncontagionist hypothesis. Both, however, conducted investigations whose thoroughness and accuracy became models of their kind. Their work was quintessentially epidemiological and it offers an uncommonly revealing view of an often complex undertaking, how one learns anything at all regarding the course of an epidemic and upon what foundations confidence in one's findings might and must stand.

François Mélier assayed epidemic yellow fever in the new French port of Saint-Nazaire and George Buchanan conducted a comparable investigation in the old Welsh city of Swansea. The northern location of these towns, given the singular ecology of the disease, was highly advantageous. Both towns, too, were relatively small and the epidemics themselves were of limited extent; these factors assured inestimable advantages in the attempt to recreate in exhaustive detail the course of an epidemic. The two epidemiologists also benefited from advances in clinical medicine and pathological anatomy: by 1860 most physicians agreed on the specificity of yellow fever. This disease was, as were other well-studied communicable diseases, a distinct clinical entity, a disease *sui generis;* it was not, as had been maintained for several generations, the ultimate and most severe stage of a series of transformable fevers.

Without the assurance of disease specificity, epidemiological inquiry quickly comes to naught. The subject of epidemiology is disease and population, not disease and the individual, yet accurate diagnosis of the individual case is the epidemiologist's necessary starting point. Clinical specificity was thus the first specificity. The second was epidemiological specificity, the fact (increasingly apparent after 1850) that each communicable disease, when correctly viewed, possesses characteristic epidemic features. That is, it exhibits traits relating especially to population and ecology that help distinguish this disease from other, similar diseases. Only later came the third and, it is believed, decisive specificity: for each such disease there exists a unique causal microorganism.

Mélier investigated in quite extraordinary detail the Saint-Nazaire yellow-fever epidemic of 1861. He then drew broad conclusions from his inquiry and devised and implemented a set of vigorous prophylactic measures for stopping the movement of yellow fever. Buchanan, too, studied his city and its epidemic of 1865 with considerable care, but it was left to his superior, one of the greatest figures in the history of British hygienic administration, John Simon, to elaborate upon the meaning of these findings. All of these investigators were working in the doctrinal shadow of the nineteenth century's most active and vocal student of yellow fever, Nicolas Chervin. Throughout the 1820s and 1830s, Chervin had assured the medical community that yellow fever was a noncontagious disease. No less important was his insistence upon the (presumed) fact that yellow fever was the product of the development of other local diseases ("fevers"), a development called forth by peculiar local or regional miasmatic conditions. Yellow fever thus could not be an exotic disease, one imported into Europe from tropical lands. A generation later, however, Mélier and Buchanan stated a conclusion that stood in flat contradiction to Chervin's claim. Yellow fever, they demonstrated, is a noncontagious disease but it is also an imported disease. This provocative conclusion posed anew the question of the origin of epidemic yellow fever and announced that the answer would be found in the connections, their nature yet to be established, between an afflicted community and a previously infected locality. Mélier and Buchanan thus dissolved the union that stood at the heart of Chervin's claims, namely, noncontagionism and the idea of local origin, and they did so using information gathered in Saint-Nazaire and Swansea. This was a step of major theoretical importance; it also held obvious implications for public health.

This book recounts the course of three epidemics of yellow fever in continental Europe and Britain. The narrative of these events, nevertheless, will be brief, for my principal purpose is not to tell a story but to analyze a process — namely, how the epidemic phenomenon in Saint-Nazaire (1861) and in Swansea (1865) was assessed — and to compare the pursuit of these investigations with the execution of a very different study carried out forty years earlier (1828) by Chervin and his associates in Gibraltar. I do not offer a general history of yellow fever, nor do I attend in a comprehensive manner to problems of disease control (i.e., quarantine and maritime inspection) or to the socioeconomic framework or consequences of disease. All of these themes will be introduced, but my principal aim is to emphasize the development of epidemiological methods and to identify the conditions that made, and make, these methods effective. The leading role in my discussion will be played by case-tracing. Case-tracing was the foundation of Mélier's and Buchanan's principal accomplishment, namely, their demonstration of how the epidemiologist could disassemble with surety and dispatch the many confused and confusing factors that contribute to the occurrence of an epidemic. From this follows their, and my, principal conclusion: epidemiological reasoning by the 1860s had acquired both autonomy and power and did so without resolving the etiological question.

I

Epidemic Yellow Fever

1

The Disease

THE SCIENCE of epidemiology was created by many hands and over many years. At the outset, epidemiologists had no settled view of either the proper subject or the limits of their new science. They agreed even less on the most appropriate method or methods an epidemiologist should employ. Nevertheless, there was agreement amidst these uncertainties that the new science would be raised upon foundations that would be assured by an assessment of the incidence and determining conditions of disease — conditions at once biological, environmental, and social in character.

This assessment presupposed the importance of analyzing numerous instances of the disease in question and of tracing, if possible, the connections between these cases. This inquiry provided fundamental data for epidemiological reasoning. Granting secure case identification (rarely an easy accomplishment) and informed circumscription of relevant determining conditions, useful conclusions might be drawn. Ideally, the epidemiologist would re-create the complete course of the disease as it moved through a discrete population. The primary concern of the medical practitioner or clinician was the individual case of disease and its management, and this focus thus had to yield to the primary epidemiological objects of inquiry, namely, disease as a population phenomenon and the many distinctive problems involved in scrutinizing and perhaps controlling an epidemic event. Close study of an epidemic offered many clues to the resolution of the fundamental problem, the mode of transmission of the disease under investigation. In some cases, it appeared that epidemiological inquiry might also offer insight into another matter of great interest, the cause of the disease. This expectation, however, was always uncertain, and epidemiologists in the era before the consolidation of the germ theory of disease were aware of, if not always responsive to, the fact that in most situations the specific cause of a given disease escaped their grasp.

During the nineteenth century, approaches to the disease phenomenon changed dramatically. Soon after 1800, British, French, and Austrian clinicians and pathologists introduced new investigative procedures and a new manner of reasoning which, taken together, placed on sound foundations a rigorous anatomicopathological or localist view of the disease process.

Their investigations ensured a new basis for the discrimination of different and previously confused diseases and for the classification of these diseases. These distinctions were now grounded on the conjunction of specific symptoms or symptom-complexes and definite, usually very localized, pathological disturbances. These advances were greatest in the resolution of the long-established category of fevers into an increasing number of very specific diseases. This was the era that defined the different forms of tuberculosis, separated typhus and typhoid fevers, and identified diphtheria.[1]

Such inquiries were singularly useful for diagnosis but did not contribute greatly to determining the cause or causes of a particular disease. With regard to communicable diseases, those which, until well into the twentieth century, imposed the greatest burden of morbidity and mortality upon society, it was not the anatomicopathological approach that suggested a solution or even a confident approach to a solution to this mystery. Here the lead was taken by laboratory inquiries, sometimes pursued in conjunction with or as a consequence of simple epidemiological study. The germ theory of disease was the product of these investigations. The germ theory offered the medical profession not only a novel view of the causal relations of several deadly and widespread diseases but conferred, by its many celebrated successes, seemingly unquestionable authority upon the experimental or laboratory approach to disease. With the rapid establishment of the germ theory after 1880, the anatomicopathological approach to disease seemed a limited, if still useful, means of inquiry. Judging by immediate appearances, the germ theory of disease conquered medicine *tout court* and in its entirety. This, at least, was the perhaps justifiable illusion on the part of the theory's advocates and even some of its critics.[2]

The role of nascent epidemiology in these movements has not been established, and my discussion addresses these questions only indirectly. I attend, instead, to what epidemiology could and could not accomplish in the absence of an assured etiological position. Not only does the timing of this study's principal events, two yellow-fever epidemics of the 1860s,

---

1. See Knud Faber, *Nosography. The Evolution of Clinical Medicine in Modern Times,* 2d ed. (New York: P. B. Hoeber, 1930), pp. 1–58; E. H. Ackerknecht, *Medicine at the Paris Hospital, 1794–1848* (Baltimore: Johns Hopkins Press, 1967), pp. 3–127.

2. But see R. C. Maulitz, "'Physician versus Bacteriologist': The Ideology of Science in Clinical Medicine," in *The Therapeutic Revolution. Essays in the Social History of American Medicine,* ed. M. J. Vogel and C. E. Rosenberg (Philadelphia: University of Pennsylvania Press, 1979), pp. 91–107. On the germ theory of disease, see Friedrich Löffler, *Vorlesungen über die geschichtliche Entwicklung der Lehre von den Bacterien* (Leipzig: F. C. W. Vogel, 1887), pp. 164–244; William Bulloch, *The History of Bacteriology* (London: Oxford University Press, 1960), pp. 155–168; K. C. Carter, "Semmelweis and his Predecessors," *Medical History* 25 (1981): 57–72.

determine this spartan approach, but the character of the epidemic disease itself allows and allowed no other conceptualization.

For no disease was ignorance of the causal agent or disagreement over modes of transmission more profound than for yellow fever. These are related but very different issues. A disease primarily of the tropical littoral of the Atlantic Ocean and of inland tropical forests, yellow fever rarely occurred in regions wholly or largely free of other serious fevers. Yellow fever was often confused with other diseases and vice versa. Yellow fever caused repeated anxiety in tropical regions, where, as one knowing observer remarked, the disease seemed "the hurricane of the human frame, equally uncertain in its recurrence, equally dark and inscrutable in its cause, equally and deplorably certain as to the reality of its existence."[3] When, on infrequent occasions, it appeared in epidemic form in Europe, it evoked public terror and social concern comparable to earlier responses to the arrival of plague and to contemporary reaction to Asiatic cholera. Between the decline of the plague in Europe after 1725 and the extraordinary arrival of Asiatic cholera on the Continent in 1830, yellow fever was feared as the supreme exotic epidemic threat to European well-being. That threat persisted until the early twentieth century, although no serious outbreaks occurred in Europe after 1880.

Yellow Fever

A European (or anyone) without previous experience with yellow fever can succumb dramatically to the disease. The French seaman Charles François Eloy, for example, arrived at Saint-Nazaire, a new French port at the mouth of the Loire River, on 25 July 1861. He had been in good health during the several weeks in which his ship, the *Anne-Marie*, had crossed the Atlantic from Havana. Once in port, Eloy supervised the unloading of the *Anne-Marie*. Late in the afternoon of Friday, 2 August, he returned to his room complaining of a sudden and severe headache, sharp pains in the upper abdomen and lower back, and generalized weakness.[4] After a tormented night, Eloy awoke on Saturday to further bodily trials. He now summoned a physician. Dr. Durand was a suspicious and shrewd observer. The extreme restlessness and anxiety of the victim were obvious to all, but Durand noted other symptoms. Eloy's eyes were inflamed; he experienced nausea and thirst; his tongue was red on the margins and tip but furred down the center line; his pulse rate was greatly elevated. Each

3. Gilbert Blane, "On the Yellow Fever," in *Select Dissertations on Several Subjects of Medical Science* (London: T. and G. Underwood, 1822), p. 316.

4. François Mélier, "Relation de la fièvre jaune survenue à Saint-Nazaire en 1861," *Mémoires de l'Académie impériale de médecine* 26 (1863): 136–138.

of these symptoms seemed much exaggerated. Comparing Eloy's singular symptoms with those of familiar local diseases, and knowing of the recent West Indian connection of the *Anne-Marie*, Durand drew a tentative yet dreaded conclusion: this was a case of yellow fever.

Eloy's situation rapidly deteriorated. His pulse now weakened and continued to fall; acute pain persisted; passage of urine slowed and then virtually stopped. Eloy's mind remained clear, yet he appeared apathetic and could speak only very briefly. His eyes and then (on the third day) his face acquired a pale yellowish tinge; this soon changed to a bold greenish yellow color. Early nausea had been accompanied by efforts at vomiting; on Sunday evening constant vomiting set in. But Eloy vomited only ingested fluids and a bit of bile: there was no indication of the copious black vomit that occasionally accompanied yellow fever and too often was held to be pathognomonic of the disease. Finally, at 4:00 p.m., on Monday, 5 August, Eloy, in total collapse on his bed, died. He had been ill for three days.

An autopsy was not performed, yet no observer entertained the least doubt that Eloy had died of a disease not customarily encountered in Saint-Nazaire or in France at large. There was, in fact, general agreement that his affliction was yellow fever, an alarming, fulminating case of yellow fever. Eloy proved to be the first victim within the city of Saint-Nazaire of the yellow-fever epidemic of 1861, and the circumstances surrounding his death and that of others in the French port will be examined more closely in the following chapters. It will be useful, however, first to describe important elements in later, largely twentieth-century additions to understanding of the character of the disease and its complex epidemic behavior. Human yellow fever has a sizable cast—a susceptible man or woman, a mosquito, and a virus—and each has its conditions of existence.

Clinical, epidemiological, and, a late arrival, etiological analyses of the disease have provided various means for the diagnosis of yellow fever. The disease is protean in its manifestations. It has been and can still be readily confused with numerous other diseases: malarial fevers; dengue fever; leptospirosis, or Weil's disease; infectious hepatitis; Lassa fever; Ebola fever; relapsing fever; and, probably often in earlier years, typhus fever.[5] Recent clinical descriptions of yellow fever present virtually the same portrait as that provided by Durand.[6] Diagnosis today is rendered more certain by chemical analysis of the blood and urine and by detection of dis-

---

5. H. R. Carter, *Yellow Fever. An Epidemiological and Historical Study of Its Place of Origin* (Baltimore: Williams and Wilkins, 1931), pp. 49–78; J. A. Kerr, "The Clinical Aspects and Diagnosis of Yellow Fever," in *Yellow Fever*, ed. G. K. Strode (New York: McGraw-Hill, 1951), pp. 413–417.

6. See the general review by Kerr, "Clinical Aspects and Diagnosis of Yellow Fever," pp. 389–425.

tinctive pathological lesions affecting the liver and kidney. If needed, and if appropriate laboratory means are available, confidence in diagnosis is given by serological tests and by isolation of the virus. Neither the celebrated jaundice nor the black vomit is present in all cases. Characteristic of a pronounced attack are sudden onset, acute and regionally localized pain (especially of head and back), and prostration, coupled with alertness and extreme anxiety. However, many infections invoke no symptoms or very mild flulike symptoms. An attack of yellow fever either causes death or confers lasting immunity upon the victim; once recovery is made, there is no recurrence of symptoms as occurs in malaria. Fever is ever-present but in itself provides no distinctive criterion for disease identification.

A disease so varied in its character elicited an equally diverse range of therapeutic measures. The fever in yellow fever naturally suggested the use of quinine, well known for its efficacy against another often devastating tropical (and temperate zone) disease, the intermittent or malarial fevers. Needless to say, quinine, which is a specific for these latter, proved to be no remedy for yellow fever. Purgation seemed to provide symptomatic relief and so did various plasters, cooling compresses, and drinks. Bloodletting, by venesection or the leech, was a common remedy. These and other measures were applied to Eloy and to innumerable others in different times and places. Whatever relief they may have given the victim, they had no perceptible effect in checking the disease. Indeed, it was recognized that no known drug or medical procedure could halt yellow fever. The disease would simply run its course. The physician's role was to assist nature, striving only to subdue painful or dangerous symptoms and maintain the bodily strength of the victim. Twentieth-century physicians offer essentially the same advice. William Osler, for example, well known for his therapeutic caution, advised that "careful nursing and a symptomatic plan of treatment probably give the best results." More recently, Albert E. Sabin, after noting that "there is no specific treatment" for yellow fever, recommended measures to secure fluid and metabolic balances within the body.[7]

Despite this continuity of therapeutic practice, knowledge regarding the disease was revolutionized between 1900 and 1930. With this new understanding, hygienic, prophylactic, and diagnostic procedures were devised that still define our essential defenses against yellow fever today. First to be resolved was a great mystery indeed: how the disease was transmit-

7. William Osler, *The Principles and Practice of Medicine*, 5th ed. (New York: D. Appleton, 1903), p. 189; A. E. Sabin, "Yellow Fever," in *A Manual of Tropical Medicine*, 3d ed., ed. G. W. Hunter, III, et al. (Philadelphia: W. B. Saunders; Tokyo: C. E. Tuttle, 1961), p. 24. See also the listing of remedies in L. J. B. Bérenger-Féraud, *Traité théorique et clinique de la fièvre jaune* (Paris: Octave Doin, 1890), pp. 770–872.

ted.[8] The long-contending advocates of contagionist and noncontagionist explanations of infectious disease divided primarily on the issues of the role of person-to-person communication of disease and the participation of environmental factors, such as an infected atmosphere or miasma, in such communication. After 1850 a number of observers began to suspect the participation of yet another actor in the yellow-fever drama, namely, the mosquito. This very small band of much-celebrated anticipators (among whom the most perceptive and insistent was the well-known Cuban physician, Carlos Finlay) pointed out that many and perhaps all of the seeming anomalies in the movement of epidemic yellow fever might be explained by positing for the mosquito an active role in moving the (unknown) causal agent from one human victim to another. Unfortunately, neither Finlay nor anyone else in the nineteenth century was able to convert this suspicion into a demonstration.

This demonstration was provided in 1900. A military medical team led by Walter Reed, who was working in Cuba following the invasion of that island by the United States Army, proved quite conclusively that yellow fever was transmitted to a susceptible human being by the bite of an infected mosquito (*Stegomyia fasciata = Aedes aegypti*). The demonstration was assured by means of human experimentation. One of the volunteers, Jesse W. Lazear, was a member of Reed's team and only the first among many investigators whose laboratory or other experimental involvement with yellow fever led to death.

The mosquito connection proved to be a critical matter in the control of urban yellow fever. The causal agent of the disease was still unknown and, as has been seen, no means existed that could halt the disease once it had taken hold in a victim. The Cuban and subsequent assaults on yellow fever were built upon a clear sense of the clinical identity of the disease and with the assistance, given the new body of knowledge, of a more complete understanding of the epidemiology of yellow fever. Knowledge of the mosquito allowed one to control an epidemic situation if one could eradicate or at least greatly reduce the numbers of this vector. Havana was the first city to be subjected to a rigorous attack on the genus *Aedes*. William Crawford Gorgas, a public health officer working under the American military administration, led the campaign to destroy the mosquito's breeding places. The peculiar ecology of the *Aedes* mosquito, which brought it in its normal round of existence into close proximity with human dwellings and hence with their occupants, greatly aided efforts to eradicate the

8. Still the most convenient if adulatory summary is H. A. Kelly, *Walter Reed and Yellow Fever* (New York: McClure, Phillips, 1906). Also A. J. Warren, "The Conquest of Yellow Fever," in Strode, *Yellow Fever*, pp. 5–37; M. D. Gorgas and B. J. Hendrik, *William Crawford Gorgas. His Life and Work* (Garden City, N.Y.: Garden City Publishing Co., 1924), pp. 68–134.

mosquito from the city. A successful campaign in Havana, where within a few months yellow fever was virtually banished from a city in which it had reigned supreme for two and a half centuries, led to further applications during construction of the Panama Canal and then as the centerpiece of a coordinated program to eliminate yellow fever from its traditional urban foci, particularly in the Americas. This was long the preoccupation of the Yellow Fever Commission of the Rockefeller Foundation, the testing place for the public health programs of that foundation and a model for other agencies devoted to international health action.[9]

The yellow-fever mosquito has occupied, too, another ecological niche, one peculiarly hazardous for the insect's coinhabitants. Conditions aboard a slow-moving wooden sailing ship allow the mosquito to prosper; if infected with the yellow-fever virus before departure, these mosquitoes could and often did create an epidemic at sea. Men and mosquitoes could also reinfect one another, a process limited only by the supply of susceptible humans and by the duration and conditions of the voyage. Moreover, since an infected mosquito remains infective throughout its life, and since its lifespan can extend over many weeks or even months, a virus-laden mosquito could enter a ship in the Americas and later attack persons in Europe who boarded the ship. The mosquito could also fly ashore and cause havoc among a population having no contact with the ship. Presumably, one or another of these chains of transmission brought yellow fever to Gibraltar, Saint-Nazaire, and Swansea, as well as to a host of other locations at other times. But in the 1820s and again in the 1860s the mosquito connection was effectively unknown. The interpretation of these epidemics and the preventive measures based upon such interpretations took form upon very different foundations.

Modern understanding of the movement of yellow fever thus depends upon the interaction of three participants: an infective agent, a mosquito, and a susceptible host. Until the early 1930s, *Homo sapiens* was generally believed to be the unique vertebrate host of yellow fever. Between 1933 and 1936, however, it was found that the infective agent could be conveyed to certain monkeys and would induce disease in these species.[10] This discovery, largely the work of Fred L. Soper and his associates, radically changed epidemiological understanding of yellow fever. It also pointed out the limits of the prevailing sanitary approach to the disease, namely, mosquito eradication. Monkey populations inhabited nonurban settings and constituted a widespread and inaccessible reservoir of yellow fever. While

9. R. B. Fosdick, *The Story of the Rockefeller Foundation* (New York: Harper, 1952), pp. 58–70.
10. See Loring Whitman, "The Arthropod Vectors of Yellow Fever," in Strode, *Yellow Fever*, pp. 231–298.

Yellow Fever: Cycles of Infection

Sylvan Yellow Fever (Central and South America and Africa)

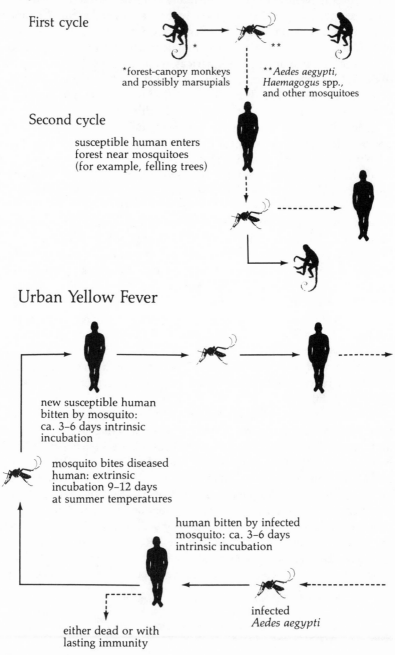

First cycle

*forest-canopy monkeys
and possibly marsupials

**Aedes aegypti,
Haemagogus spp.,
and other mosquitoes

Second cycle

susceptible human enters
forest near mosquitoes
(for example, felling trees)

Urban Yellow Fever

new susceptible human
bitten by mosquito:
ca. 3–6 days intrinsic
incubation

mosquito bites diseased
human: extrinsic
incubation 9–12 days
at summer temperatures

human bitten by infected
mosquito: ca. 3–6 days
intrinsic incubation

infected
Aedes aegypti

either dead or with
lasting immunity

control of urban yellow fever remained both possible and effective, there could now be little thought of global eradication of the disease. Nonurban or, as it came to be called, jungle or sylvan yellow fever, persisted independently of man, striking the latter only when forest-dwelling humans chanced to come into contact with the infected mosquitoes that ordinarily occupied the forest canopy. The felling of trees proved and proves to be the most common moment of contact.

Another major discovery in these years led to protective immunization, which, when joined by constant surveillance and sustained antimosquito measures, provides the foundation for present-day protection against yellow fever. As early as 1902, Walter Reed and James Carrol had voiced the hypothesis, based on their experimental observations, that the determinative agent of yellow fever was a virus. Not until 1928, however, when Adrien Stokes, J. H. Bauer, and N. Paul Hudson provided extensive confirmatory evidence for the viral hypothesis, could this fundamental etiological issue be resolved.[11] Within a decade, this discovery had been exploited to devise procedures for inducing effective artificial immunity against the disease. These inquiries led, too, to the development of sophisticated serological tests to be used for diagnostic purposes and for study of the incidence of yellow fever in human populations.

There is, in short, nothing simple about the biological and epidemiological character of yellow fever. The disease involves several primate hosts, with man being the principal party in urban yellow fever but usually only an accidental victim in jungle yellow fever. In common with many other severe viral diseases, the transmission of yellow fever requires an insect host, and here several species can be involved. Yet, despite occasional sus-

11. Walter Reed, and James Carroll, "The Etiology of Yellow Fever: A Supplemental Note," *American Medicine* 3 (1902): 301–305; Adrian Stokes et al., "The Transmission of Yellow Fever to *Macacus rhesus:* Preliminary Note," *Journal of the American Medical Association* 90 (1928): 253–254; Max Theiler, "The Virus," in Strode, *Yellow Fever,* pp. 41–163. Also W. A. Sawyer et al., "Vaccination against Yellow Fever with Immune Serum and Virus Fixed for Mice," *Journal of Experimental Medicine* 55 (1932): 945–969; K. C. Smithburn, "Immunology," in Strode, *Yellow Fever,* pp. 203–227. More recent developments in understanding the disease are concisely portrayed by W. G. Downs, "History of Epidemiological Aspects of Yellow Fever," *Yale Journal of Biology and Medicine* 55 (1982): 179–185. Now the entire nucleotide sequence of yellow-fever viral RNA has been sequenced: C. M. Rice et al., "Nucleotide Sequence of Yellow Fever Virus: Implications for Flavivirus Gene Expression and Evolution," *Science* 229 (1985): 726–733; also T. P. Monatu, "Glad Tidings from Yellow Fever Research," ibid., pp. 734–735. Yellow fever has been banished from many of its haunts but only by means of careful attention to travelers, regular individual and occasional mass vaccination, and close sanitary surveillance. Nevertheless, a threat persists, not least because (uninfected) *Aedes* mosquitoes have reestablished themselves in favorable ecological situations and in close association with man; see Jonathan Leonard, "The Ghost of Yellow Jack," *Harvard Magazine* 83 (1981): 20–27.

picions, the very notion of disease transmission by means of a nonverte-
brate vector did not enter the mainstream of medical and epidemiological
thought until the 1890s, primarily through Theobald Smith's startling demonstration that Texas cattle fever was caused by a tick-borne protozoan.

A disease in its totality should be viewed as a human construct, an
intricate combination of many objectively described features bound together by a perceived deleterious effect, the latter working against the observer himself or against his domesticated animals and cultivated plants.
The well-portrayed set of apprehensible yellow-fever characteristics, namely,
the symptoms formed into a clinical entity, were clearly defined by the
1850s and have not been substantially modified since that time. Despite
this, the disease is largely a creation of the twentieth century. Causal agent,
nonhuman hosts, the characteristic ecology of these hosts and how the
latter determines contact with the human host—all of this information is
now deemed crucial, yet none of it was known prior to 1900. But, as the
following discussion will reveal, epidemiology before this date was not
powerless when confronted by yellow fever.

It is important to distinguish between what an investigator hoped to
accomplish and what was actually accomplished. Among the many essential elements of an epidemiological investigation, some elements could be
determined with confidence and others, although constantly brought to
the fore, simply could not be resolved. In 1865, for example, few physicians concerned with the problems of communicable disease failed to
speculate on the specifically etiological question, the causal agent of the
disease. For yellow fever, this passionate endeavor never yielded more than
idiosyncratic personal satisfaction, if even that. August Hirsch, medical
geographer without peer and a physician whose knowledge of infectious
disease was well-nigh exhaustive, remarked derisively in 1883 that "Hypotheses as to the *nature of the yellow fever poison,* leaning sometimes
to one side, sometimes to the other, have exhausted the ingenuity of the
profession without advancing our knowledge a single step."[12] Constant
dispute arose, too, regarding contagionism and noncontagionism, again
without awarding clear victory or even sustained, if precarious, satisfaction to either party.

In a sense, consideration of contagion and its modalities, or rumina-
tion on the identity of a hypothetical etiological agent, raised broader questions. Here one touched near fundamental yet seemingly unanswerable
questions about the nature of the disease, its cause, and how, precisely,
this cause is conveyed to a susceptible human being. Yet behind these con-

12. August Hirsch, *Handbook of Geographical and Historical Pathology,* 3 vols., trans.
from the 2d German edition by Charles Creighton (London: New Sydenham Society, 1883–
1886), 1:369.

troverted matters, phrased here in a reductionist manner, there were important epidemiological questions that could be resolved, given a willingness to concentrate upon specific aspects of particular epidemic situations. Answers to these questions depended upon exacting local inquiry and open-mindedness with regard to contested etiological issues. It was within this deliberately circumscribed framework that François Mélier, exploring epidemic yellow fever in Saint-Nazaire in 1861, and George Buchanan, working in Swansea in 1865, reached a new and more useful understanding of the epidemic behavior of the disease. Both remained noncontagionists, yet each realized that that interpretation asked new questions as well as answered old ones. Each adopted, and defended with ample, cogent, and reliable observations, the view that yellow fever in nonendemic regions is an imported disease, not one that results from changed local conditions. Importation in turn posed fundamental questions about the use or abandonment of traditional preventive measures, notably quarantine or other forms of border control. The reality of importation of disease led to a return to favor, and systematic application of, carefully designed sanitary control measures. Neither Mélier nor Buchanan failed to consider the etiological issue. Nonetheless, the true force of their respective inquiries depended, as each recognized, upon what should be viewed as a more specifically epidemiological investigation, upon the exhaustive tracing of yellow fever within discrete populations. And it was these investigations, not speculation upon the causal agent, that led to definite and, it appears, effective hygienic action.

European Contacts

The origin of yellow fever is lost in the obscurity of time and in the varied turns of scholarly controversy. Claims for a West African and a tropical American origin have been made, with the African-origin hypothesis remaining seemingly the stronger contender. The question is really twofold. The first part asks when yellow fever first manifested itself in a particular locality. But a meaningful response to that question depends upon an acceptable answer to the second part: when and how was this disease recognized as being a distinct entity, one which was in fact yellow fever and not in whole or in part but an aspect of any of the numerous other diseases with which confusion was so easy and frequent? In his remarkable study of the history of yellow fever published in 1931 (thus before the discovery of jungle yellow fever), Henry Rose Carter had to begin with these questions, seeking trustworthy criteria by which to evaluate reports and claims reaching back some four hundred years.[13]

13. See Carter, *Yellow Fever,* passim. Not all epidemics will be accurately identified and

A further general concern deserves emphasis. However the African- or American-origins dispute be resolved, yellow fever from the outset posed a scientific problem only to a third set of observers, namely, European military men, clergy, administrators, and physicians. Human experience with the disease no doubt long antedates European contact with it. Varied biological evidence (widespread immunity and a diversity of vectors) suggests that what Europeans came to call yellow fever was established in West Africa long before that region was approached by European explorers in the fifteenth and sixteenth centuries. Africans do not possess an innate immunity to the disease, but those populations living in infected areas first touched by European seafarers surely enjoyed a high level of protection, presumably an immunity acquired during childhood when the disease is relatively less severe. (Childhood mortality due to yellow fever might, nonetheless, have been high.) The Europeans possessed no such immunity and the result was usually disastrous. West Africa, however, also presents other fevers, notably severe malarial fevers, with some of which the Europeans had had equally little or no medical experience. Confusion of diseases and epidemics was inevitable, and because of this it seems less remarkable that the earliest confident identification of yellow fever in Africa dates only from 1782.

By this time, however, the disease had been active in the Americas for well over a century.[14] Carter concludes that the earliest authenticated American epidemic occurred in the Yucatan in 1648; the following year yellow fever appeared in Havana, a city whose name later became synonymous with the disease. Epidemics occurred sporadically thereafter throughout Central and northern South America. By 1700 yellow fever had entered North America, sweeping as far north as New York. In the later eighteenth century, and particularly after 1790, the Atlantic and Gulf coasts of the new United States joined the West Indies and Central America as the favored targets of the disease.

In the Americas, too, the matter of paramount importance was the presence of sizable nonimmune, that is susceptible, populations. These were the native Americans and immigrant and transient Europeans. The existence of a significant resident European population in the Americas, whether civilian or military, made all New World fevers a matter of keen medical

---

many will pass unnoticed. Sources of confusion are numerous, ranging from the diverse symptomatology of the disease to the character of the written records in which the trace of yellow fever is being sought.

14. J. J. Pedersen, "The Antiquity of Sylvan Yellow Fever in the Americas" (Los Angeles: Ph.D. diss., University of California, 1974), presents evidence questioning the African-origins view and favoring the presence of the disease in the Americas well before the mid-seventeenth century.

curiosity and concern, the physicians in question being European in origin and training. The African coast sheltered no such exotic population; there were few military personnel and traders. Their stays were often brief, usually ending as a consequence of chronic ill health or an early death, with fever being the leading cause of death. Larger numbers of Europeans moved into tropical Africa beginning only in the nineteenth century, and those numbers were small compared with the European conquest of the American continents and peoples. In Africa, only physicians with the army and, especially, the navy seriously concerned themselves with the epidemic character of the region, and they did so usually in episodic manner.[15] These physicians learned a great deal. However, because of the sustained presence of the disease in the Americas and the continuing appearance in American cities of fresh susceptibles from the homeland (or from unaffected inland regions), "European" contact with yellow fever was initially and preponderantly that which was established in areas of European settlement in the New World.

Yellow fever in Central and tropical South America became, as no doubt it was already in Africa, an endemic disease. It moved sporadically from community to community, its spread doubtlessly checked by the fluctuating supply of human susceptibles but probably encouraged by the peculiar ecology of the rising sugar economy.[16] In certain unfortunate cities, such as Havana, Guayaquil, and Rio de Janeiro, each a center of major population movements, yellow fever settled in with man and could reappear year after year. European observers in America and American physicians thus had ample opportunity to examine the disease firsthand.

Indeed, today much of the best-known literature dealing with the history of epidemic yellow fever recounts events in North America. Repeated onslaughts of yellow fever along the Gulf and Atlantic coasts of the United States provoked lengthy and contentious discussion of the disease, its putative cause, and its epidemic behavior. Certain yellow-fever epidemics in

15. See S. F. Dudley, "Yellow Fever, As Seen by the Medical Officers of the Royal Navy in the Nineteenth Century," *Proceedings of the Royal Society of Medicine* (United Services Section) 26 (1932): 443–456. Alexander Bryson provides an evocative account of the varied experience with the disease in his *Report on the Climate and Principal Diseases of the African Station; Compiled from Documents in the Office of the Director-General of the Medical Department, and from other Sources* (London: William Clowes, 1847). Also David Scott, *Epidemic Disease in Ghana, 1901–1950* (London: Oxford University Press, 1965), pp. 26–64; L. J. Bruce-Chwatt and J. M. Bruce-Chwatt, "Malaria and Yellow Fever," in *Health in Tropical Africa during the Colonial Period*, ed. E. E. Sabben-Clare et al. (Oxford: Clarendon Press, 1980), pp. 43–62; D. G. Carlson, *African Fever. A Study of British Science, Technology and Politics in West Africa, 1787–1864* (Cambridge, Mass.: Science History Publications, 1984).

16. J. D. Goodyear, "The Sugar Connection: A New Perspective on the History of Yellow Fever," *Bulletin of the History of Medicine* 52 (1978): 5–21.

the United States exercised a profound influence on medical theory and professional organization. They caused serious economic disturbances and elicited widespread, if not long-enduring, demands for the creation of strong local and even national public-health authorities. Particularly notorious were the epidemics in Philadelphia in 1793 and New Orleans in 1853 and, above all, the staggering epidemic in Memphis in 1878.[17]

These and other lesser epidemics were mass affairs, focused upon sizable urban areas and involving cities in which population movements were extensive. For example, at the time of the epidemics in New Orleans and Memphis, migrants heading for unsettled lands in the central and western United States were rapidly passing into and through those cities. Large-scale nineteenth-century American yellow-fever epidemics were not propitious settings for an exhaustive and consistent analysis of the many parameters of the epidemic phenomenon. The need for medical management of the disease was always urgent and commanded many resources. Central investigatory authority was either absent or was only constituted during the course of the epidemic. But, above all, large areas and large and highly mobile populations made it exceedingly difficult to resolve the critical issue, the tracing of each several case and determining the connections between cases or between these cases and presumably relevant local conditions. To compound the problem, yellow fever occasionally visited the same location in successive years; this behavior raised still other perplexing questions. Presumably, these analytical difficulties also arose when yellow fever struck urban areas in Central and South America, and they definitely confused the investigation of the great Barcelona epidemic

17. See, for example, J. B. Blake, "Yellow Fever in Eighteenth-Century America," *Bulletin of the New York Academy of Medicine* 44 (1968): 673–686; C.-E. A. Winslow, *The Conquest of Epidemic Disease* (Princeton: Princeton University Press, 1943; reprint, Madison: University of Wisconsin Press, 1980), pp. 193–235; J. H. Powell, *Bring Out Your Dead. The Great Plague of Yellow Fever in Philadelphia in 1793* (Philadelphia: University of Pennsylvania Press, 1949). Also John Duffy, *Sword of Pestilence. The New Orleans Yellow Fever Epidemic of 1853* (Baton Rouge: Louisiana State University Press, 1966); T. H. Baker, "Yellowjack. The Yellow Fever Epidemic of 1878 in Memphis, Tennessee," *Bulletin of the History of Medicine* 42 (1968): 241–264; T. L. Savitt, *Medicine and Slavery. The Diseases and Health Care of Blacks in Antebellum Virginia* (Urbana: University of Illinois Press, 1978), pp. 240–246; D. B. Cooper, "Brazil's Long Fight against Epidemic Disease, 1849–1917, with Special Emphasis on Yellow Fever," *Bulletin of the New York Academy of Medicine* 51 (1975): 672–696. Also idem, *Epidemic Disease in Mexico City, 1761–1813: An Administrative, Social and Medical Study* (Austin: University of Texas Press, 1965), pp. 155–182. The frequency and distribution of New World yellow-fever epidemics may be seen in the tables and discussion in Hirsch, *Handbook of Geographical and Historical Pathology* 1:318–328, and Bérenger-Féraud, *Traité de la fièvre jaune*, pp. 23–199. A tour de force of exposition and criticism is René La Roche, *Yellow Fever, Considered in its Historical, Pathological, Etiological, and Therapeutic Relations*, 2 vols. (Philadelphia: Blanchard and Lea, 1855).

of 1821, Europe's first experience with truly overwhelming urban yellow fever.

Highly localized and short-term outbreaks of yellow fever did occur in the New World. These could be and were closely analyzed, and they sometimes yielded information of fundamental epidemiological importance. Carter, for example, observed yellow fever in two small Mississippi towns. He concluded that a definite period (roughly two weeks) elapsed between the appearance of the first case or cases and that of secondary cases. This clearly indicated an extrinsic incubation period, and Carter offered this conclusion on the eve of Reed's discovery of the role of the mosquito.[18] Perhaps nowhere, however, did yellow fever present itself so clearly and distinctly, and nowhere did an epidemic of the disease proceed in so conspicuous a manner (i.e., where both the beginning and end are sharply marked and contacts are thoroughly exposed), as in regions where the disease rarely, if ever, established itself. Such was the case in northern Europe.

Contemporary observers understood well the analytical advantages of the small, isolated epidemic. One need only compare the report made of the great New Orleans epidemic and that prepared a decade later by Mélier, describing events in Saint-Nazaire, to appreciate these advantages.[19] It is possible that the story I relate in the following pages could also be recovered from American sources. I am not aware that this effort has ever been made and I am confident that the inquirer's task would be more difficult than mine has been. It is likely, too, that the American setting, given the ecology of this singular disease, would render the conclusions from such an assessment far more ambiguous than those which may be drawn from events in Saint-Nazaire and Swansea.

European students of yellow fever nonetheless owed a great debt to their American colleagues. From the earliest Western contact with the disease, the physician who never set foot outside of Europe had gained his basic fund of description and interpretation of yellow fever from publications by colleagues who resided or had visited across the sea. This was especially true after yellow fever assumed a central role in what may be called a growing epidemiological consciousness, a product of experience and doctrinal conflict in the 1790s. But, as is so often the case with infec-

18. H. R. Carter, "A Note on the Interval Between Infecting and Secondary Cases of Yellow Fever From the Records of the Yellow Fever at Orwood and Taylor, Miss. in 1898," *New Orleans Medical and Surgical Journal* 52 (1900): 617–622: cited in A. L. Bloomfield, *A Bibliography of Internal Disease. Communicable Diseases* (Chicago: University of Chicago Press, 1958), p. 496.

19. E. H. Barton, *The Cause and Prevention of Yellow Fever at New Orleans and Other Cities in America*, 3d ed. (New York: H. Baillière, 1857).

tious diseases, one needed only to wait. It was merely a matter of time before yellow fever came to greet the European physician in his homeland.

The disease was, in fact, reliably reported to be present in Europe even before it was recognized in Africa, a reminder of the Europocentric perspective of its observers. As expected, the cities of the Iberian peninsula were struck first and most frequently. Here both climate — a long and very warm summer and autumn — and established trade connections requiring frequent sailings — joining especially the entrepôt of Havana with Spain and Brazilian ports with Portugal — favored the importation and nurture of exotic diseases. It was and is difficult to be sure that a given past epidemic was in reality an epidemic of yellow fever. Hirsch accepted the presence of the disease in Cádiz in 1700 and on several additional occasions during the eighteenth century. Pedro Francisco da Costa Alvarenga, in writing of the Lisbon epidemic of 1857, claimed, however, that yellow fever first appeared in Europe in Lisbon in 1723.[20] These were reports of local epidemics, instances in which the disease spread through the urban (and perhaps rural) population and was not confined to the appearance of ailing or convalescent sailors who had just disembarked from a transatlantic ship (the latter being a not unusual event).

Until the 1790s yellow fever was confined to these outbreaks plus that at Málaga in 1741. Century's end, however, brought rapid change. The increase of yellow fever in Europe was no doubt tied to an increase in maritime activity, both commercial and military. An epidemic that had begun in Cádiz in 1800 had spread by 1804 to Cordoba, Grenada, Valencia, and into Catalonia. Gibraltar, too, was seriously attacked. Yellow fever thereafter returned repeatedly to southern Spain. These lesser epidemics then culminated in the terrible Barcelona outbreak of 1819–1821.[21] The disease subsequently returned to Spain (Barcelona, 1870; Madrid, 1878) and to Gibraltar (1828), but without the catastrophic consequences of 1819–1821.

Portugal suffered somewhat later. Minor epidemics may have followed that of 1723, but it was during the 1850s that serious damage was done. Oporto and Lisbon were infected. The 1857 epidemic in the latter city was awesome in both scale and mortality, a comparable if unwelcome partner to the Barcelona epidemic of 1821.

Occasionally yellow fever escaped from the Spanish ports or was

20. Hirsch, *Handbook of Historical and Geographical Pathology* 1:335–337; P. F. da Costa Alvarenga, *Anatomie pathologique et symptomatologie de la fièvre jaune qui a regné à Lisbonne en 1857*, trans. P. Garnier (Paris: J. B. Baillière, 1861), p. 2.

21. See G. D. Sussman, "From Yellow Fever to Cholera. A Study of French Government Policy, Medical Professionalism, and Popular Movements in the Epidemic Crises of the Restoration and the July Monarchy" (New Haven: Ph.D. diss., Yale University, 1971), pp. 46–152.

perhaps conveyed directly from America to other parts of Europe. Two thousand persons were reported stricken in Livorno, Italy, in 1804; perhaps one third died of the disease. Smaller outbreaks occurred at Brest in Brittany in 1802 and 1856; in Southampton in 1852; in the city and environs of Saint-Nazaire in 1861; and in Swansea and neighboring areas in 1865. Surely the most unusual, because it was the most remote epidemic of yellow fever in Europe (if the disease was in fact yellow fever), was that reported to have struck Dublin in 1826.[22]

With the exception of the Lisbon epidemic of 1857, the Gibraltar epidemic of 1828 was the last major European outbreak of yellow fever. As I shall attempt to show (in chapter 2), scrutiny of the Gibraltar epidemic, while conducted by many hands and in seemingly exhaustive detail, led only to renewed disputes on virtually every front. Clinical and pathological identity, definite connections between cases, appropriate therapies, and epidemiological and etiological implications were all left unresolved. To public authorities and to many physicians, Gibraltar came to be seen as a lesson in reverse: this was no way to conduct an investigation or to establish the essentials of an epidemic. This was particularly true of those matters that concerned the critical issues of local origin or importation and upon which not only interpretation but action depended.

It is easy enough to criticize one or another conclusion drawn by the Gibraltar physicians or to attack the methods employed in their investigations. However, faced with the epidemic phenomenon of the 1830s, it is today abusive — and in 1830 was surely impossible — to propose more efficacious or more reliable methods or to articulate more objectively grounded conclusions. Gibraltar marks a definite point in the evolving study of epidemic yellow fever and provides a basis for comparison in the present volume. Some forty years later, European epidemiologists had occasion again to examine the disease on their homeground.[23] In particular, Mélier and Buchanan appreciated and fully exploited the singular opportunities

22. R. J. Graves, "Yellow Fever of the British Islands," in *Clinical Lectures on the Practice of Medicine*, 2 vols., 2d ed., ed. J. M. Neligan (Dublin: Fannim, 1848) 1:280–302.

23. This was the generation that first began systematically to use the term *epidemiology* and its derivative *epidemiologist*. The former was probably introduced by the lexicographer, historian, and philosopher Emile Littré. A new entry in Nysten's classic dictionary read: "Epidémiologie. Recherches sur les causes et la nature des épidémies. L'épidémiologie est une part importante de l'histoire de la médecine, attendu que les maladies se sont éteintes, d'autres se sont transformés, d'autres enfin apparaissant nouvelles." Emile Littré and Charles Robin, eds., *Dictionnaire de médecine, de chirurgie, de pharmacie, des sciences accessoires et de l'art vétérinaire de P. H. Nysten*, 11th ed. (Paris: J. B. Baillière, 1858), p. 515. The context for this coinage was the distinctive "historical pathology" then current, especially in Germany: see Johanna Bleker, "Die historische Pathologie, Nosologie und Epidemiologie im 19. Jahrhundert," *Medizinhistorisches Journal* 19 (1984): 33–52.

afforded by the locations and conditions of Saint-Nazaire and Swansea. In each case a distinct disease, recognizable as yellow fever, occurred in a town where the normal disease situation was known and where, at the moment of the epidemic, disease levels were low. New means of communication assured rapid and continued inspection of the epidemic scene almost from the moment of onset. Saint-Nazaire stood relatively isolated from other parts of France and Swansea was near no major metropolitan area. In both communities, each case of disease could be identified and each one was traced. Mélier and Buchanan well understood how to translate these general conditions into distinct advantages. Importation was their common conclusion. Furthermore, the specific conditions allowing importation could be determined, remedial measures were proposed, and, in France, imposed. In Mélier's case, at least, we have a striking illustration of the adage of the right man being in the right place at the right time. It should be added that while place and time were largely fortuitous, the man and especially the capacities of his science were well prepared for such an eventuality.

Three Epidemics

Epidemiological method writ large probably knows no limits. The problem to be resolved dictates the methods to be employed: case-tracing, laboratory diagnosis, field investigation, statistical analysis, numerical modeling, and so on. The character of the disease also determines which method or approach is to be borrowed or indeed invented for the occasion. For the following discussion, the desire and the capacity to trace exhaustively each case of yellow fever in Saint-Nazaire and in Swansea, and the failure to do so in Gibraltar, are matters of highest importance. Case-tracing is the fundamental element in early epidemiological method. The conditions necessary for success in this difficult art were early recognized.

The French physician Esprit Gendron worked in the tradition of his master, Pierre Bretonneau, who was an accomplished rural epidemiologist as well as an outstanding clinician. In 1834 Gendron noted concisely the basic desiderata for conducting an effective epidemiological investigation:

> For the physician who desires to make himself useful, without question the most important study he can undertake is that of epidemics. When epidemics attack large cities or entire provinces, when they spread over various regions of one or several nations, then the concern of leaders of science or the administration is awakened. But in the midst of these ailing multitudes, of these decimated populations, the physician, no matter how skillful he be, [always]

arrives too late to be able to trace the epidemic to its starting point and to discover under what circumstances the various victims have been attacked. He who in good faith seeks the truth will find that such difficulties do not exist in isolated places of small size. With a bit of perseverance, one can almost always find the initial victim. Knowing thus the point of departure of the epidemic, the observer can record the conditions that seem to determine its advance. . . . Living as I do in a small town and practicing in the countryside, I have followed epidemics in miniature and I shall speak above all of what I have seen.[24]

These words constitute a credo for the aspiring epidemiologist; they offer a research program and the conditions necessary for its success.

By discovering the first case in an epidemic, the investigator gained an indispensable *terminus a quo*. Then, if other cases could be reliably connected to this first case, the bonds of that connection could be explored. To the epidemiologist these bonds were the subject of greatest interest, for it was precisely here that the determining conditions of the movement of communicable disease might be identified. Here, too, a basis might be established for control of the epidemic. Gendron's remarks reveal, however, that one could not expect to conduct such an inquiry amidst a large and confused urban epidemic, the traditional preoccupation of European physicians who studied mass disease. What was needed was a limited epidemic, limited in duration surely but above all limited in reach over space and population. Lastly, yet a matter of supreme importance, there was the promise to report only what had actually been seen, a promise which, when kept, demanded minimally the early and continued presence of the investigator at the scene of the epidemic.

In examining three nineteenth-century yellow-fever epidemics, my aim is to exhibit central features of early epidemiological investigation and to display the character of the science in its doing. For this purpose, events at Saint-Nazaire and Swansea in the 1860s move to the fore. The inquiry at Gibraltar forty years earlier affords a perspective for viewing the two

24. Esprit Gendron, "Recherches sur les épidémies des petites localités," *Journal des connaissances médico-chirurgicales*, no. 7 (1834): 193. A half-century later one of the greatest of all epidemiologists voiced the same opinion. Rudolf Virchow, in expressing his views on the contested issue of the cause and transmission of Asiatic cholera, declared in 1885: "I place greatest value, however, on the precise determination of certain, especially conclusive cases or small groups of cases. . . . A small but well observed and well established set of individual cases is for me much more decisive than a whole series of large epidemics. The latter I can know only in broad outline and in no way can I analyse their particularities." Virchow, in "Conferenz zur Erörterung der Cholerafrage (Zweites Jahr)," *Deutsche medizinische Wochenschrift* 11, no. 37A (1885): 31. The classic modern statement favoring study of the small epidemic is W. N. Pickles, *Epidemiology in Country Practice* (Bristol: John Wright, 1939).

later investigations. Gibraltar was, within Gendron's meaning, a small world and one whose epidemic situation might, it would appear, have been thoroughly apprized. But it was not, and the effort to do so seemed only to have revitalized the battle between conflicting doctrines. The contagionists, although already on the defensive, did not capitulate before the new evidence assembled on the Mediterranean; noncontagionists claimed to have won a scientific victory, yet their triumph was really more secure in the political and administrative domain.[25]

In France, then still the European leader in matters of hygiene, discussion of the meaning of the Gibraltar epidemic followed immediately upon review of the hygienic implications of the Barcelona epidemic and led to important changes in sanitary practice. Gibraltar strengthened the demands of Nicolas Chervin, the leading apostle of noncontagionism, to reduce or virtually eliminate sanitary control over the nation's frontiers. During the 1830s France gradually disassembled such measures; loosely put, she abolished quarantine. In the aftermath of the Saint-Nazaire epidemic it became clear that this behavior was both extreme and fatal, and during the 1860s France began rapidly to reconstruct administrative and medical means to protect herself from invasion by exotic communicable disease.

Preventive measures thus again seemed to have merit. Very early in the yellow-fever disputes, Gilbert Blane, an English naval physician, observed that yellow fever, "like all others of a pestilential or malignant nature, sets at defiance the art of physic in its curative capacity; human skill, of which the most anxious and judicial exertions have not been wanting, has been found of little avail in abating the fatality of this epidemic. The great, and only substantial source of hope to be looked to must consist in preventive measures." Blane recognized, however, that "from some peculiar circumstances in the nature and character of this disorder, there has most unfortunately been much difference of opinion, whether it is the subject of prevention, for great doubts have arisen in the minds of many whether it is contagious."[26]

Naturally, any consideration of prevention turned first to the question of the cause of the disease. Regarding yellow fever this was not only unknown, but it seemed unknowable. With the benefit of twentieth-century hindsight one can see that the major part of the celebrated contagionist-noncontagionist dispute over yellow fever was due to total ignorance of the third participant, the mosquito. With human yellow fever, the notion

25. Gibraltar's role as the essential reference point for the yellow-fever battles of the early nineteenth century was emphasized in the pioneering discussion by E. H. Ackerknecht, "Anticontagionism between 1821 and 1867," *Bulletin of the History of Medicine* 22 (1948): 562–593.
26. Blane, "On the Yellow Fever," p. 285.

of causation necessarily embraces two nonhuman terms, a viral agent and an arthropod vector. Causation thus demands consideration of both the pathophysiological changes that ensue when the virus meets a susceptible host and the whole range of issues that surround the transmission of that virus from one human being to another. Nineteenth-century research could not solve the former riddle, involving both the identification of a supposed microscopical agent and the discovery of measures to counteract the malign influence of that agent. With regard to the question of transmission or the epidemiological component, much, in fact, was done, and done in complete ignorance of the role played by the mosquito. Using increasingly thorough epidemiological means, certain features of the disease could be explored in new ways. Decisions could be reached that profoundly affected an understanding of the movement of the disease. Above all, it could be shown in a conclusive manner that, whatever the particular nature of its causal agent, yellow fever was indeed brought about by an agent that was transported from one locality to another. Yellow fever was not a local product, arising *de novo* from the filth or fouled air of a town or region or by the transmutation of a less severe fever. It was a specific disease whose cause was presumably a specific miasma, the movement of which could be traced in detail. This tracing could lead to at least one important conclusion regarding causation, namely, continuity of cause.

Furthermore, however the causal question be resolved, it is evident that the sick individual provided the irreducible datum for the epidemiologist. But this victim was only a starting point, not the issue itself. The key to the new science was the disease phenomenon as represented by an assemblage of sick individuals. The epidemiologist did not, however, deny the work of the medical practitioner. He presupposed this work, and then sought to transcend the clinician's viewpoint in his quest to understand disease as a population phenomenon.

Once again, the epidemics at Saint-Nazaire and Swansea were, within Gendron's meaning, limited epidemics confined to small areas. Mélier and Buchanan capitalized upon this fact. They traced every recognized case of yellow fever in their respective communities and ascertained and evaluated every conceivable parameter that might have affected the movement of the disease. These two towns were seen to offer virtual laboratory conditions. They constituted nature's own experiments, in which all pertinent factors appeared to be clearly defined and susceptible to exact description. They lent themselves well to the formulation of novel and important conclusions.

One must not conclude, however, that Mélier and Buchanan answered satisfactorily all previously posed questions. Their respective conclusions, and those added by John Simon to Buchanan's discussion, were not in agreement on many points. Moreover, certain of their conclusions would later be modified or replaced, and some were altogether rejected. The significance of their work is truly the manner in which they conducted their inquiries. Their practice may have been imperfect, yet, when contrasted with the manner in which the Gibraltar epidemic of 1828 was examined, that practice is singularly illustrative of the development of epidemiological methods over a period of approximately forty years. By the 1860s these methods had been often and well tried. When they were turned to yellow fever in localities in northern Europe, their power was greatly enhanced by the characteristic ecology of these regions. In a meaningful sense, the events at Saint-Nazaire and Swansea, having called forth their investigators, offered each an uncommonly propitious setting for study. In turn, their work provides an unusually clear insight into the development of epidemiological method and practice.

2

Gibraltar, 1828

IN 1828 YELLOW FEVER had not yet entered metropolitan France. French observers, nonetheless, had good reason to be concerned about the disease. Within the previous quarter century, yellow fever had repeatedly attacked sugar islands in the French Antilles. In a convincing display of its fatal power, it had destroyed the large army sent by Bonaparte to Haiti to reduce the forces of the independent-minded Toussaint L'Ouverture. British and Spanish interests, too — and soon thereafter the interests of the newly independent Central and South American states — were no less affected by yellow fever, the latter by its continuing role in tropical life and death and the former by the presumably real, yet still unmeasured threat that it posed to Europe itself.

The reality of a threat to northern Europe was made most clear, however, by the Barcelona epidemic of 1821. French and English observers now recognized that yellow fever might in fact move further, and northward, within Europe. French civil and medical authorities understood particularly well that the hundred miles separating Barcelona and Perpignan offered a very narrow barrier to the entrance of the disease. It seemed evident, too, that from this important coastal trade route a connection might be established with inland France.

Yet close proximity was only one among the many features of the Barcelona epidemic that disturbed France and other European nations. More alarming was the scale and cost in lives of this unprecedented disaster. Yellow fever first appeared in Barcelona in August 1821 and disappeared only during the following winter.[1] The incidence of the disease

1. The major report on the epidemic is Victor Bally et al., *Histoire médicale de la fièvre jaune, observée en Espagne et particulièrement en Catalogne, dans l'année 1821* (Paris: Imprimerie royale, 1823). An opposing view was expressed by J. A. Rochoux, *Dissertation sur le typhus amaril, ou maladie de Barcelone, improprement appelée fièvre jaune* (Paris: Béchet jeune, 1822). For context and widespread implications, the fundamental study is G. D. Sussman, "From Yellow Fever to Cholera. A Study of French Government Policy, Medical Professionalism, and Popular Movements in the Epidemic Crises of the Restoration and the July Monarchy" (New Haven: Ph.D. diss., Yale University, 1971), pp. 46–152. Also L. F. Hoffmann, *La peste à Barcelone. En marge de l'histoire politique et littéraire de la France sous la Restauration* (Paris: Presses Universitaires de la France, 1964).

was never assessed and even mortality remained a matter for speculation or rough estimation. The lowest estimates suggest that five thousand died; other estimates raise the number of dead to twenty thousand. The population of Barcelona was itself uncertain but probably stood somewhat above one hundred thousand. Yellow fever during the six months of the active epidemic thus took the lives of between 5 and 20 percent of the urban population.

The French government dispatched official observers to Barcelona whose reports tended to confirm the claim that yellow fever was an imported disease. The observers claimed that yellow fever was passed from person to person; it was therefore a contagious disease. But there were counter-reports that strongly favored a noncontagionist interpretation, the cause of the epidemic being assigned to local environmental conditions. In the following year, 1822, Nicolas Chervin entered the dispute, creating a turning point in public and professional discussion of the disease. He did so just as the French government promulgated the first comprehensive law (on 3 March 1822) that imposed both system and seeming rigor upon the theretofore chaotic sanitary defense of the nation's frontiers. The stage was thus set for a singular battle that raged for some forty years. While the argument seemed mostly a matter of medical doctrine, it also involved important political and economic interests.[2]

The epidemiological and hygienic issues raised by the Barcelona yellow-fever epidemic were kept alive by Chervin's campaign against the implementation of the new sanitary law. It was only too clear that the several investigations of the recent Spanish epidemic had neither resolved any outstanding questions regarding the nature or mode of transmission of the disease nor proposed widely acceptable and effective protective measures to combat it. What did occur was a polarization of French medical opinion. When epidemic yellow fever again touched European shores, now in Gibraltar in the summer of 1828, there was hope for a definitive response to at least some of these questions. This expectation was rapidly deceived.

The Gibraltar epidemic was closely observed from the outset by British military and Spanish civil physicians residing on the peninsula. Their inquiries led to no settled conclusions; indeed, their disagreements were as marked as those that arose amongst the members of the official French investigatory commission. It was the latter investigators, however, who, having joined forces with the British, produced the principal account of the epidemic. This group also attempted to provide an analysis of the movement of the disease through the military and civilian populations.

2. E. H. Ackerknecht, "Anticontagionism between 1821 and 1867," *Bulletin of the History of Medicine* 22 (1948): 562–593.

The Gibraltar Commission

For a multiplicity of discordant facts and an abundance of opposed opinion, stated in intransigent and often inflammatory manner, few medical events can match the discussions provoked by the yellow-fever epidemics of the early nineteenth century. Gibraltar in 1828 was no exception. Public authorities in France were fully aware of the problem. Recognizing the importance of studying an epidemic firsthand, they made a valiant attempt to appoint a balanced and sensible commission to be sent to the peninsula. The three commissioners were selected by the Academy of Medicine, a quasi-official body, and went to Gibraltar under the auspices of the French government. In choosing the three commissioners, all parties wished to avoid the charge that these Gibraltar investigators, like those sent earlier to Barcelona, had been selected simply to reaffirm the contagionist view of yellow fever. This charge was expected to come from critics of the Bourbon administration, as well as from the noncontagionist camp, but its being raised was nicely avoided. Such was the circumspection of the Academy and of the government, and such the nature of the evidence collected, that the Gibraltar commission refused to offer in its collective name any conclusions at all. The individual commissioners, however, were free to speak their minds and one of them repeatedly did so.

Nicolas Chervin (1783–1843) had returned to Europe from America late in 1822.[3] He then learned of the Barcelona epidemic and of the report on its character being prepared by French physicians. He immediately set off for Catalonia, determined to inquire whether a distinct disease had in fact been present in Barcelona and whether its cause had been imported or was to be sought in the local sanitary situation.

Chervin had received his medical training in Paris (M.D. 1812) and soon thereafter had gone to America. There his interest in yellow fever was evoked which, in later life, became an obsession. Between 1815 and 1822 he traveled widely in North America and the Antilles, collecting medical opinion regarding three essential features of the disease. Is yellow fever, he asked, imported into the Americas? Is it confined to particular localities? Does it spread by means of person-to-person contact? He answered these questions, respectively: no, generally yes, and no. From these seemingly well-established conclusions he then erected a major argumentative structure directed against contagionism.

Chervin observed much yellow fever, but for the most part he posed questions to practitioners who had worked closely with victims of the disease and had followed its epidemics. On his death bed, he summarized

---

3. François Dubois d'Amiens, "Notice historique sur M. Chervin," *Mémoires de l'Académie royale de médecine* 12 (1846): xxxvii–lix.

his life's mission: "I have nothing to leave [to anyone]. All that I received from my parents and all that I have earned in practice has been devoted to the investigations regarding the origin and mode of propagation of yellow fever that I have pursued for twenty-six years. This I did with the aim of modifying the sanitary practices employed against this disease on the European continent."[4] Chervin's reflections on the Barcelona epidemic and his much publicized views regarding yellow fever in the Americas rendered him a well-known public figure. Chervin represented the noncontagionist and nonimportationist positions on the commission. Unlike his fellow commissioners, he also possessed extensive firsthand experience with yellow fever.

The other commissioners had at this time apparently never seen a case of the disease.[5] It seemed important that one member enter the fray without known preconceptions. For this role, Pierre Charles Alexandre Louis was chosen. Louis (1787–1872), the great pathological anatomist at l'Hôpital de la Charité, was a man accustomed to accumulating facts and a person who was thought to let such facts speak strictly for themselves. Louis possessed vast clinical and pathological experience — in association with others he performed some five thousand postmortem examinations during his career — and was known to approach generalization with caution. That caution was best expressed in his celebrated introduction of the so-called numerical method into medical reasoning. Louis was deemed to be the neutral party on the commission. To represent the contagionist viewpoint, a disciple of Pierre Bretonneau was chosen. Armand Trousseau (1801–1867) was to become in the 1840s the most brilliant clinical teacher in France. He began his career in Paris in 1822 and was there the enthusiastic spokesman for Bretonneau's overtly biological view of the etiology of communicable diseases. It seemed to many that this young man would favor the contagionist viewpoint and thus balance Chervin's inflexible noncontagionism. The happy symmetry of these choices was, in fact, meaningless. Louis ventured only a brief and contradictory opinion regarding the cause of the disease and Trousseau, by no means a rigid contagionist, long remained silent regarding this question. Chervin, however, eagerly exploited the vast documentation gathered in Gibraltar, using it to further the noncontagionist outlook and its sanitary implications.

In sending out his commission, the Minister of Interior probably real-

4. Ibid., p. lvi.
5. Jules Béclard, "Notice sur la vie et les travaux de Pierre-Charles-Alexandre Louis," in *Notices et portraits* (Paris: G. Masson, 1878), pp. 227–257; idem, "Éloge de M. Trousseau," *Mémoires de l'Académie impériale de médecine* 29 (1869–1870): clxxiii–cxcii. William Pym and David Barry represented British interests on the commission, but only Barry participated in the investigation.

ized that its members would never sufficiently agree on doctrine to be able to propose new or spread old dogma. They could, however, be trusted to bring home abundant and perhaps well-authenticated facts, these collected by the commissioners themselves. They were instructed, in short, to gather information and eschew opinion. This they did, but the available data posed insuperable analytical problems.

The report of the commission, tersely titled *Documens recueillis par MM. Chervin, Louis et Trousseau,* was by far the most substantial account of the Gibraltar epidemic.[6] The work was published in 1830 and represented the combined efforts of a joint French and British inquiry. The *Documens* is a singular work. It reported in varying detail the course of 597 cases of sickness that occurred in Gibraltar between August and December 1828. A brief introduction was provided but a conclusion was not.

Organizing their report in short sections or "documents," the commissioners attempted to establish a common plan of analysis for each case or set of cases. There was a presumption that all were cases of yellow fever, but it is apparent that this was not so. The name and address of the person or persons afflicted were recorded, and the number and relationships (familial or casual) of other persons in the same household were given. An effort was made to establish the date of onset of the disease and to record its progress to either recovery or death. Often symptoms were reported *in extenso,* the commissioners knowing only too well the serious implications of deciding whether yellow fever was a distinct disease entity or only the heightened form of other and perhaps rather common fevers. Confusion of diseases, however, did occur. The commissioners tried to pay particular attention to connections, real and potential: connections between households; between members of a given housing unit; between persons wherever found when one or more in the chain had succumbed to yellow fever; between sickness, housing, and serious local sanitary disorders such as improperly sited cesspools, poorly maintained sewers, and fouled streets or housing. Lastly, the commissioners sought to determine whether any victims of the Gibraltar epidemic had previously suffered from yellow fever. This was no easy matter to decide and usually remained moot. Uncertain diagnosis and the unsure meaning of "slight" cases of fever during this and previous epidemics in Gibraltar made this question, like so many others, often unanswerable.

The commissioners did, however, succeed in avoiding the presentation of conclusions of any kind. Surprisingly, given Louis's presence on

---

6. *Documens recueillis par MM. Chervin, Louis et Trousseau, membres de la commission française envoyée à Gibraltar pour observer l'épidémie de 1828; et par M. le Dr. Barry, médecin des armées anglaises,* 2 vols. (Paris: Imprimerie royale, 1830).

the commission, not even a numerical summary of cases and mortality was provided. The authors of the *Documens* also scrupulously avoided overt discussion of the two issues that were of supreme popular and sanitary interest and administrative concern: cause/transmission (contagion or noncontagion; importation) and appropriate public action (quarantine or unrestricted access to ports). Clearly, the documents were offered as the facts of the matter; the reader, like each of the authors, was left to draw his own conclusions.

In normal years Gibraltar was a reasonably healthy locality. A contemporary survey of the health conditions of the town indicated that the winter months posed no uncommon hazards and in the summer and early fall, when heat and humidity reached their peaks, only various "bilious and putrid disorders" became threatening.[7] These struck newcomers with especial violence. Frequent cases of intermittent and other fevers, measles, scarlatina, pulmonary disturbances, and—a singular local problem— elephantiasis or bucnemia, provided the disease background against which regular seasonal upswings or truly epidemic outbreaks had to be measured. This was, however, only a generalized qualitative portrait and it made no reference to the situation in any given year, including the summer and fall of 1828.

Yellow fever was a familiar visitor to Gibraltar. The most recent serious epidemic had occurred in 1814, and that of 1804 had been of major proportions. Cases were numerous and death was common; survivors acquired immunity. During the six months when this latter epidemic raged, 1,082 members of the British garrison (officers, soldiers, women, and children) died; total mortality from all causes amongst the same group during the preceding twenty-four months was only 91.[8] Overall mortality in Gibraltar in 1828 was high and yellow fever was a major factor. Bulletins issued by local authorities reported that 5,383 persons fell ill with fever or serious disease. Of these, 1,183 died, all from what was called yellow fever.

Indicative of the problem facing epidemiological assessment of this epidemic was the uncertainty regarding such numbers.[9] David Barry, a Brit-

7. John Hennen, *Sketches of the Medical Topography of the Mediterranean: Comprising an Account of Gibraltar, the Ionian Islands, and Malta; to which is prefixed a Sketch of a Plan for Memoirs on Medical Topography*, ed. J. Hennen (London, 1830), pp. 92–119.

8. Ibid., p. 98.

9. Reported by P. C. A. Louis in his *Anatomical, Pathological and Therapeutic Researches on the Yellow Fever of Gibraltar of 1828. From Observations taken by himself and M. Trousseau, as Members of the French Commission at Gibraltar*, trans. from the manuscript by G. C. Shattuck (Boston: Charles C. Little and James Brown, 1839), p. 259. This work was subsequently published in the original French: "Recherches sur la fièvre jaune de Gibraltar de 1828," *Mémoires de la Société médicale d'observation* 2 (1844): 1–299.

ish observer, independently reported that 5,543 cases of "epidemic disease" occurred between August and December 1828 and of these 1,631 died.[10] Louis argued that the number of persons reported ill by the public authorities was surely too small; during a serious epidemic persons with mild cases avoided making themselves known for fear of being forcibly transported to hospital or *lazaretto*. Because of this, the case-fatality rates reported by the authorities, 22 percent, and by Barry, 29 percent, were surely too high. Louis published his own figures only a decade later. These were drawn from the cases studied by the French commission and they thus presumably reflected a more assured population, one that had survived the peak of the epidemic. These data indicated a case-fatality rate of 15.4 percent.[11] Implicit in all of these figures is the suggestion that all or most of these cases *were* cases of yellow fever.

The French observers concluded that the first victim of the Gibraltar epidemic was Mary Testa, who became ill on 21 August.[12] She was a resident of the Twenty-fourth District, thought by many to have been the focus of the epidemic; her case was also the first to be presented in the *Documens*. Information regarding the next 596 cases was collected over a four-month period (December 1828–March 1829), that is, long after the beginning and peak of the epidemic. The commissioners prepared and attempted to follow a standardized set of questions (unfortunately, these were not published with the edited responses); this, surely, is a mark of Chervin's influence. The questions were submitted to individuals, families, physicians, and municipal and military authorities. From each was requested a circumstantial report regarding his or her experience with the disease. Perhaps 10 percent of the afflicted population was reached in this manner.

10. Reported in [Chervin], "Lettre sur l'épidémie de fièvre jaune qui a regné à Gibraltar dans l'automne de 1828, et sur les opérations de la commission envoyée par le Ministre de l'Intérieur pour observer cette maladie; adressée par M. le docteur Chervin, l'un des membres de cette commission, à M. le docteur Monfalcon à Lyon," *Transactions médicales* 1 (1830): 74n; David Barry, "On the Gibraltar Epidemic of 1828," *London Medical and Physical Journal*, n.s., 10 (1831): 93.

11. Louis's use of his figures poses a difficulty. He declared (*Researches on the Yellow Fever of Gibraltar*, p. 259) that mortality among the "600" (that is, 597) cases for which the commission made reports was in "the proportion of 1 to 6-½" or 15.4 percent; this would indicate that the number of deaths within this group was 92. Elsewhere (ibid., p. 283), however, he stated that the number of persons dead of yellow fever was 76, case fatality now falling to 12.7 percent. There is no way to reconcile these figures with one another or with the death rate (22 percent) based on the public bulletins.

12. Louis, too, accepted this widespread conclusion but he also reported (ibid., pp. 356–359) that Diego Ansoles, a gardener, had fallen ill on 16 August and died a few days later; almost certainly his was a case of yellow fever. Yet this was stated to be a "sporadic" case, that is, one that occured, as seemed to happen, between genuine epidemics. Ansoles was not to be, therefore, the first victim of the 1828 epidemic.

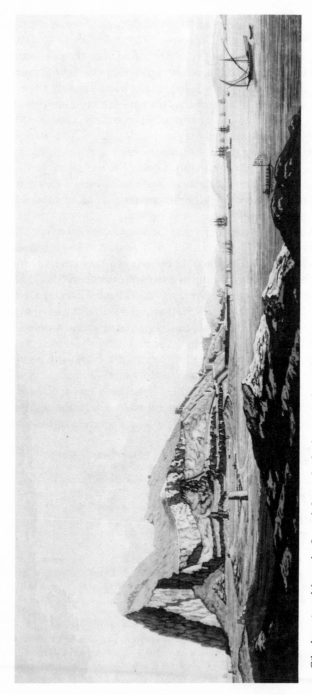

Gibraltar viewed from the Spanish Lines. In the foreground stretches the unoccupied *terrain neutre*. In the middle distance the Old Mole, around which stood most shipping in the port, including the *Dygden* and the *Méta*. Behind lies the precipitous and dry Rock of Gibraltar. (Courtesy of the Trustees of the British Museum.)

32

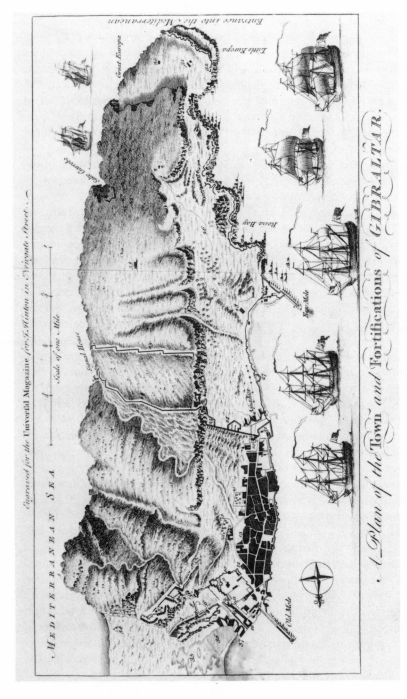

Engraved for the Universal Magazine for L. Hinton in Newgate Street.

MEDITERRANEAN SEA

Scale of one Mile

Entrance into the Mediterranean

A Plan of the Town and Fortifications of GIBRALTAR.

The Rock of Gibraltar, with the town and port in the lower left. To the left (north) the *terrain neutre*; below, the small and densely occupied settlement adjoining the port between the two moles. (Courtesy of the Trustees of the British Museum.)

33

With Louis and Trousseau acting as secretaries, the responses were then edited, reorganized, and placed in the *Documens* in rough order by town district and other localities. In each report of a case or a group of cases an effort was made to determine a set of general or special conditions that prevailed prior to the occurrence of the case or cases in question. The several and diverse conditions thus recorded established the character of the inquiry and, as may be expected, also established the range of possibilities amongst which one or another explanation of the epidemic might be sought.

This approach suggests that case-tracing was an important goal of the commissioners. Certainly they realized the significance of assaying in detail the conditions surrounding an epidemic — conditions such as physical setting, sanitary ambience, and human contacts. But the circumstances of the Gibraltar investigation did not permit this: available evidence permitted no assured conclusions. As was so often the case in studying epidemic yellow fever, the numerous, varied, and changing connections between local conditions and healthy and diseased individuals (and also those between diseased persons and other individuals) could not be seized. Confusion and contradiction ensued. As always, each inquirer was free to select the evidence that seemed best to fit his needs and to reject or, more commonly, ignore all else.

Events in the Flat Bastion Road, the most seriously affected part of the Twenty-fourth District, illustrate these problems.[13] Illness, presumably yellow fever, had struck the home of the Serfatis (personal names were reported only occasionally). Martin, who lived nearby, had a clerk who visited the Serfatis; the daughter of this clerk fell "ill." (Was it yellow fever? The commissioners offered no opinion.) Martin also had a domestic who carried instructions to the clerk (nothing was said of where they met); she, too, fell "ill." The Francis family maintained regular communications with their neighbors, the Serfatis. Mr. and Mrs. Francis had had yellow fever during a previous epidemic and did not become ill in 1828; the other thirteen members of their household had had no previous experience with the disease. On 3 September, one of the Francis daughters was stricken with "black vomit"; she died on the fifth. That child had been quickly isolated and, somewhat later, the various members of the family were dispersed to other parts of Gibraltar. By October, nevertheless, all of the children had taken ill, two seriously, but only the one child died. An aunt who had tended that child, thus remaining in intimate connection with her, became very ill. Another child, who had been sent away before she could have close contact with her ailing sister, returned home after six weeks

13. *Documens recueillis par MM. Chervin, Louis et Trousseau* 1:1–15.

and in excellent health. Within ten days, however, she too was sick and exhibited all the symptoms previously seen in the dead child.

By 3 September, when Francis's daughter took ill, most houses along Flat Bastion Road already contained much sickness. One could view this acknowledged fact as highly suggestive of the contagious character of the disease. The French commissioners made no comment at all. It was conventional wisdom in 1828 that the presence of a foul smell during an epidemic indicated the likely presence of a poisonous miasma. One must look to the atmosphere. This the commissioners did, but they found that sewer and other smells in the Flat Bastion Road in August 1828 seemed normal for the season and were scarcely perceptible within doors. Still, Francis did report that an overwhelming odor of "rotten flesh" had prevailed when his daughter fell ill.

Save for the sorrowful comment by the commissioners that they could not determine if Serfati had had any connection with his neighbor Mary Testa, the supposed original victim of the epidemic, the above description embraces the full reach of this instance of the documentary material gathered by the French physicians. From such evidence assured conclusions could not be drawn. The many victims in the Francis family, for example, might show the untoward effects of an unknown contagion, moving from person to person. But there was nothing to deny the possibility that, since all lived under the same vitiated atmosphere, an infective miasma had been active, its presence made evident by the foul smell that at least one concerned person reported to have reigned at the onset of the epidemic. It may be noted, too, that these seemingly authenticated facts, scrupulously recorded by astute investigators, were gathered from recollections related over four months after the events in question.

The perils of late oral reporting are marvelously illustrated by the case of Charles Kelly. Kelly had arrived in Gibraltar about 1 July. His ship, the *Méta*, may well have carried yellow fever. Kelly himself appeared "yellow" to one observer. He was also reported to have stated that he had been ill during the crossing from Havana and that one or two fellow crew members had died at sea. In early August Kelly's friend Leakey visited the *Méta*, which he found to be a very clean ship, but thereafter he, too, fell seriously ill.[14] The *Méta* had other connections ashore. Kelly was said to have given his laundry to Mr. Whitelark, who passed it on to Mrs. Pepin; her husband was reported "dead," but there was no knowledge of when and how he died. The captain of the *Méta* had his laundry done by Mrs. Thomp-

14. Ibid., pp. 32–37. The commissioners, reporting symptoms secondhand and well after the event, agreed that Leakey had died of yellow fever. But those symptoms — high fever and much sweating, but no pain or vomit, and full recovery after only three days — suggest a malarial fever, not yellow fever.

son. Mr. Thompson had had yellow fever in 1804; Mrs. Thompson caught the disease in 1828 but only "long after" doing the captain's laundry. Mrs. Whitelark did no ship's laundry but did become ill. So did her children, and Mr. Whitelark himself died of yellow fever.[15]

These tangled and utterly inconclusive reports become even more confused when the words of Mrs. Gordon are heard. She knew Kelly personally and found him to be healthy after his voyage. Her husband visited the *Méta* often and apparently suffered no ill effects. Mrs. Gordon, who was seeking a place aboard the ship for her son, spoke with the captain of the *Méta* and reported that she had heard directly from him that there was no place for the boy because the ship's "crew had remained unchanged" since leaving Scotland for Havana and then returning across the Atlantic to Gibraltar.[16]

Kelly thus was reported to have said that two men had died on board the *Méta* between Havana and Gibraltar, and death is a biological event not likely to deceive even the medically untutored eye. The ship's captain, however, was reported to have said that no men had died aboard his vessel for an even longer period of time. There was, of course, no way to reconcile this contradictory testimony. The commissioners, arriving months after the events in question, spoke with neither Kelly nor with the *Méta's* captain, both of whom had long before vanished into parts unknown. The French investigators thus contented themselves with reporting without comment opposing opinion, from which neither they nor anyone else could draw useful conclusions.

Yellow fever in Gibraltar also offered countless instances of the kind of evidence that assured the continued prosperity of the contagionist-noncontagionist disputes, the following being only a few examples. Edward Acres reported that he had had no contact whatsoever at home, at work, or aboard a ship with persons who in any manner had been ill with yellow fever or with objects that had been in contact with sick persons. Alas, he was stricken by the disease.[17] José Hernandez, by contrast, returned in September from the temporary evacuation camp on the *terrain neutre* to the infested Twenty-fourth District. There he had stayed with and treated his daughter, a yellow-fever victim. Upon his later return to the camp and despite the fact that he neither took precautions nor changed his clothes, Hernandez completely escaped the disease.[18] In the one case,

15. Ibid., pp. 37–40. In this case, Whitelark's symptoms strongly suggest yellow fever: sudden and severe headache and backache, jaundice, black vomit, delirium, and epistaxis, leading to death in five days.

16. Ibid., p. 142.

17. Ibid., p. 41.

18. Ibid., pp. 45–46.

sickness resulted without any personal contact; in the other case, close personal contact did not spread the disease. Perhaps mere physical proximity was not dangerous. But then one might cite the case of the children of Francisco Matos. These children followed their parents into new quarters that were located near rooms where death from yellow fever had earlier occurred.[19] The children, having entered these rooms, soon took ill with the disease. Similarly, the niece and children of Crooks lived exposed to a narrow courtyard desperately fouled by the stench from an ill-tended privy; they contracted yellow fever.[20] The noncontagionist rejoiced in such facts, just as the contagionist could find doctrinal solace in the spread of yellow fever through the Francis family.

This kind of evidence was the common coin of epidemics and epidemiology before 1850. The problem arose with numerous epidemic diseases, with Asiatic cholera and epidemic typhoid fever as well as with yellow fever. Taken at face value, such evidence might point in many directions, but it could give sure priority to none. With regard to yellow fever, for example, available facts seemed to disallow the necessity of personal contact for the transmission of the disease. This had long been the critical negative argument of the noncontagionist and it remained so. In those few cases where contagion, that is, genuine person-to-person transmission, seemed to have occurred, the absence of a controlled situation always permitted the noncontagionist to escape the dilemma by pointing out that the chain of victims all lived under the same local conditions, presumably a poisonous local atmosphere. But that argument only invited the traditional contagionist rejoinder: why did not *all* or most persons experiencing that atmosphere, and perhaps *all* or many localities within the region suffering from the same maleficent climatic condition, contract yellow fever? The disease was epidemic but by no means did it touch all persons, including many who surely had had no previous experience with it. Local conditions alone obviously did not suffice to generate or spread the disease.

The Case of the *Dygden*

The preponderance of evidence in the *Documens* pertained to yellow fever within and between the different districts of Gibraltar. The epidemic remained localized — it did not spread to nearby Spain and apparently did not travel further aboard the many ships that touched at Gibraltar late in 1828 — and those who studied its behavior attended principally to local conditions. This was consistent with the noncontagionist view that such

19. Ibid., pp. 84–86.
20. Ibid., pp. 88–90.

conditions lay at the root of the disease. But this was not, obviously, the only possible explanation. There were others who held that yellow fever was not indigenous to Gibraltar and must therefore have been introduced onto the peninsula. To these observers, introduction by sea, genuine importation from an afflicted and most probably a tropical land, seemed the most promising explanation of the origin of the epidemic. This hypothesis demanded scrutiny and did receive some desultory attention. But here the evidence proved singularly deficient, now being more sparse and unreliable than even that which had been gathered for the town and garrison.

The French commissioners understood the importance of trying to determine the circumstances under which the supposed first victim took sick. This was Mary Testa. Falling ill on 21 August, she remained in serious condition until 9 September and then gradually recovered. As far as could be determined, she had remained within the Twenty-fourth District and had had no direct contact with either the Spanish frontier or with the other foreign element in the life of Gibraltar, namely, the frequent commercial and naval shipping in the harbor.[21]

Direct contact no, but indirect contact there had been. Mary Testa's brother was a maritime or sanitary guard. It was his responsibility to board and remain with those ships entering the port that local authorities wished to place under sanitary surveillance. On 27 July he boarded the *Dygden,* a Swedish ship that had arrived several weeks earlier from Havana and had already discharged her cargo.[22] Testa slept aboard the *Dygden,* which at the time stood out in the harbor, and he returned home to his sister and family on 6 August. He had not been sick on the ship and was not ill when he went ashore. (He did become ill, however, on 9 September, perhaps with yellow fever.) He had not returned home empty-handed. The commissioners remarked that he brought with him his bedding, blanket, and soiled clothing. Moreover, the captain of the *Dygden* was reported to have visited Mary Testa on 13 August, perhaps to leave clothing for washing; Mr. Testa's own washing had been done by Maria de la Conception, who did not become ill. The commissioners were unable to determine if Mary Testa had had the disease before. She was cared for by her two sisters, neither of whom became ill. She received numerous visitors and also went visiting when she was again able. Only one of her contacts, other than her brother, was known to contract yellow fever and that occurred at the end of September.

Obviously, if Mary Testa was the first victim and thus the starting point for the subsequent spread of the epidemic, it was of capital importance

21. Ibid., p. 1; 2:366.
22. Ibid., 2:367–369.

to know what the medical experience of the *Dygden* had been. This the commissioners could not learn; they had arrived much too late.[23]

The *Dygden* had left Havana on 12 May and reached Gibraltar on 28 June. She was placed in quarantine upon arrival, her bill of health (*patente*) being deemed unacceptable. She then remained moored in the harbor until free communication with shore (*pratique*) was permitted on 6 August. The exercise of quarantine had not been unduly rigorous or atypical. Sanitary guards came and went and the *Dygden's* cargo was brought ashore during July.

With regard to epidemiological method, the interesting question is how the French commissioners gathered details concerning events aboard the *Dygden*. They did not examine the ship, for it had departed months earlier. They posed no questions to captain or crew, for they, too, had left Gibraltar long before. They could put no questions to port authorities, for the latter had kept no record of these matters. Instead, they interviewed anyone they could find who had had contact with the ship or its personnel. Testa himself reported that the *Dygden* seemed a very clean ship. He saw no illness aboard and no men who seemed convalescent. He nonetheless had the ship "purified" by washing hammocks and mattresses and airing the sails. The commissioners also learned that the captain of the *Dygden* had sworn to port officials upon entrance into the harbor that the "denghey" (dengue fever) had reigned in Havana at the time of his ship's departure (this being the cause of the *Dygden's* unacceptable bill of health) and that, in crossing, two men of "delicate health" had died, probably from excessive labor and not from fever of any kind.[24] He obviously made no comment about the possibility of "denghey" or yellow fever, two easily confused diseases, appearing amongst the crew while at sea. While the ship was in quarantine a second sanitary guard (Nicolas Montano) was aboard with Testa, but no one in his family was reported to have taken ill. (There is no indication, however, that the commissioners interviewed him.) Lastly, it was noted that at least one other ship, also from Havana, was in port at the same time as the *Dygden*. Of this ship the commissioners could say absolutely nothing, although it is probable that it was the *Méta*.

The commissioners faced an impossible task. Even if they had wanted to examine importation as a serious explanation, which seems unlikely, they could not do so in the only truly effective manner. The ship had sailed, and with it had vanished the primary personnel and physical evidence the commissioners might have hoped to interview or examine. But they did

23. The commissioners' full report on the *Dygden*, ibid., pp. 366–376.
24. Ibid., pp. 368–369.

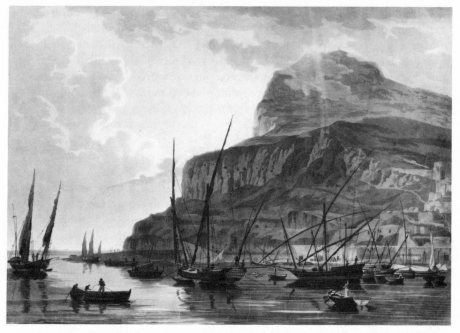

View from the west of the peak of Gibraltar and, below, the major line of fortifications facing toward Spain and the northern perimeter of the town. In the foreground, the port for local shipping lying just north of the Old Mole. (Courtesy of the Trustees of the British Museum.)

trace and speak with a number of local men who had worked aboard the *Dygden* while she was in port and who had sailed with her on a short run to Cádiz. With one exception these men reported a clean ship, no bad odors, a healthy crew, and no rumors of prior serious illness. The exceptional informant, Manuelo Garé, declared, however, that the *Dygden* offered the worst smells that he had encountered in twenty-five years at sea and that the crew seemed "pale and weak." Testimony even further removed from the events was given by a Mrs. Ballardo, who reported an earlier conversation with an unnamed man previously in her employ who had gone to sea and had sailed aboard the *Dygden* from Havana to Gibraltar. He revealed to her that he had been seriously ill in Havana. After two weeks in the hospital he boarded the *Dygden.* En route to Gibraltar he observed that two men died and that they had displayed an unspecified "fever." Apparently no one asked him whether others on board had been ill at sea or were sick upon arrival at Gibraltar.

These comments and observations constitute the entire presentation by the commissioners of the events surrounding the *Dygden* and, in fact, regarding shipping in general at Gibraltar in 1828. Obviously, such facts could not and did not offer secure grounds for drawing meaningful conclusions regarding the importation or nonimportation of yellow fever. The situation in Gibraltar's harbor was, simply put, quite beyond reconstruction. Romaine Amiel, a British army surgeon who witnessed the epidemic, made this clear. An Army Medical Board inquiring into the epidemic posed this question: "What vessels arrived at the port during the period of the two years specified [1827–1828], as extracted from the harbour master's or health officer's register?" Amiel replied:

> It has been impossible to obtain the returns called for from the offices mentioned in this query; and all that has come to my knowledge is, that the number of vessels arrived in this bay from the Transatlantic countries, where the yellow fever usually prevails, since the year 1816, to the breaking out of the late epidemic, amounts to eight hundred and forty four.[25]

Perhaps these records were merely unobtainable, perhaps they simply had not been kept, but it is a fact that none of the reports on the epidemic, whether lengthy (the French *Documens*) or brief (articles by Amiel, Barry, and others), provided even a rudimentary record of shipping at Gibraltar during the summer of 1828. Amiel's figures, no more than an aggregate of shipping over twelve years, indicate that on average five or six ships from the Americas entered Gibraltar each month. But late summer and early fall marked the peak of the sugar shipping season and surely many more than the average number of ships reached Gibraltar at this time, several of them coming from Havana. Chervin, Louis, and Trousseau, however, remarked only two among these ships, the *Dygden* and the *Méta*, and provided only minimal information regarding their condition and experience.

Chervin Triumphant

The major conclusion to emerge from analysis of yellow fever at Saint-Nazaire and Swansea was that the disease, or, more precisely, its cause, had been imported into those towns. The manner of importation, too, could be stated with reasonable assurance. François Mélier and George Buchanan reached these conclusions by means of careful study of the arrival and activity of ships in the two ports and by tracing in detail the movement of persons in relation to those ships. They sought and found reliable data

25. Romaine Amiel, "Answers to Queries from the Army Medical Board on the Epidemic at Gibraltar 1828," *Edinburgh Medical and Surgical Journal* 35 (1831): 259.

by which to test and, as they discovered, confirm the importationist hypothesis.

Importation and nonimportation here assume an epidemiological significance equal to the accustomed interpretive categories, contagionism and noncontagionism. There is, and was, no simple equivalence between these two sets of options. The importationist could be and often was an adherent of the noncontagionist doctrine; such was the case of Mélier and Buchanan. Noncontagionism in other hands, however, might assign exclusive etiological importance to changed local conditions and spurn the thought of importation of an exotic cause of communicable disease. Such was Chervin's tenaciously held position.

The 1830s and 1840s were the years of Chervin's triumph and also of greatest prosperity of doctrinaire noncontagionism. The Gibraltar epidemic had followed immediately upon the celebrated discussion by the Academy of Medicine, and an ensuing uproar in the medical press, of Chervin's wealth of documentation concerning yellow fever in the Americas.[26] After 1828, his publications constituted a running commentary on the general problem of disease transmission. His subject was yellow fever, and his work supplied, often in astonishing form, a set of conclusions such as the *Documens* had failed to provide. He it was who made public the supposed lessons of the Gibraltar epidemic.

Chervin denounced the claim that yellow fever had reached Gibraltar aboard the *Dygden*. Here was a silly notion, one based on a "multitude of absurd and ridiculous tales" and whose only result was to show that the importationist hypothesis was "without any foundation" whatsoever. Furthermore, he confidently observed, "in my view, and I believe, in that of every impartial and unprejudiced person, there exists not the faintest hint of proof that the yellow fever that ravaged the [Gibraltar] garrison last autumn [that is, autumn 1828] was of exotic origin."[27]

Chervin assigned the origin of the disease to strictly local factors. These

26. This massive report, the work of a committee of eighteen, announced the Academy's conversion to noncontagionism and its rejection of the contagionist conclusions of its own investigators sent to Barcelona only six years earlier: [G. B. A. Coutanceau], *Rapport lu à l'Académie royale de médecine, dans les séances des 15 mai et 19 juin 1827, au nom de la commission chargée d'examiner les documens de M. Chervin, concernant la fièvre jaune* (Paris: Firmin Didot, 1827). Ackerknecht, "Anticontagionism between 1821 and 1867," pp. 575–582, shows how the failure of sanitary cordons and quarantines to check the spread of Asiatic cholera contributed greatly to the prosperity of the noncontagionist cause. The character of Chervin's American inquiries, and also the possible bias in his approach, is well portrayed by M. J. Waserman and V. K. Mayfield, "Nicolas Chervin's Yellow Fever Survey, 1820–1822," *Journal of the History of Medicine* 26 (1971): 40–51.

27. [Chervin], "Lettre sur l'épidémie de fièvre jaune . . . adressée par M. le docteur Chervin, à M. le docteur Monfalcon," pp. 65, 66.

included exhalations from fouled sewers and cesspools, crowded and filthy housing, and a steady west wind which held all of this tainted air over the upper town. With an eye on the contagionist theory, he took care to recite the host of cases in which close or repeated personal contact failed to transmit the disease. He also noted that in Gibraltar, night exposure in isolated places by persons who had had no contact with diseased individuals had produced the worst cases. The heavy night air was singularly dangerous.[28]

Chervin stated the principal claims of the rival etiological theories in a fair and full manner but, as the following words reveal, there could be no question as to which proposition he held to be true. "At this time," he observed,

> there are only two major medical views regarding the origin and character of yellow fever: that of the *contagionist* and that of the *infectionist* [noncontagionist]. According to the former, this disease results from a *virus*, a miasma, a germ or a principle of whatever kind which arises and is developed within the sick individual. It then serves to spread the affliction amongst healthy persons, either by direct or indirect contact or by means of the air over a short distance.
>
> The infectionists hold, on the contrary, that yellow fever originates in an altered, vitiated or contaminated atmosphere. The exhalations generated by decomposing vegetable or animal substances, this [process] being encouraged by a high temperature and probably also a distinctive atmospheric situation and by other causes of which we are ignorant, are the responsible agents. Yellow fever never results from the mere presence of sick individuals. These persons we can bring together and can touch in any conceivable manner under all sorts of conditions and yet there is no danger of contracting yellow fever in so doing. Finally, all we need to do to avoid the disease is to escape from the infected atmosphere, for the disease is never seen to trespass beyond the limits set by its [atmospheric] cause.[29]

28. [Chervin], ibid., pp. 67–68. If, Chervin added, all of these causes prove unsatisfactory, we still have that "quid divinorum" upon which, like Hippocrates before us, we can fall back. Indeed, anything but contagion.

29. Chervin, *Examen des nouvelles opinions de M. le docteur Lassis, concernant la fièvre jaune, ou réponse à la brochure que ce médecin vient de publier sur les causes des épidémies en général, et plus particulièrement de celle qui a régné, l'an dernier, à Gibraltar* (Paris: J. B. Baillière, 1829), pp. 5–6. Following René La Roche (*Yellow Fever, Considered in its Historical, Pathological, Etiological, and Therapeutical Relations*, 2 vols. [Philadelphia: Blanchard and Lea, 1855], 2:236 ff.), I have throughout employed the terms *noncontagion* and *noncontagionism*. Better, perhaps, would be the traditional terms, used by Chervin, *infection* and *infectionism*, for these describe the positive character of his view. But common usage seems to favor *noncontagionism* or its equivalent, *anticontagionism*. I avoid the latter only because it places stress on the etiological dichotomy, not the epidemiological context, and is also peculiarly associated with the polemics of the 1820s and 1830s. Ackerknecht ("Anticontagionism

The contagionist position was then denounced as being the "religion of the administration," a reference to the long-standing and close association between contagionism and the justification of sanitary surveillance of national frontiers. Chervin knew that the noncontagionist view favored the removal of such controls. The practical consequence of the new disease theory was to support freedom of movement, particularly unhindered movement of ships at sea and in ports. It is this conjunction of medical theory, economic expectation, and political agitation that placed Chervin at the center of the antiquarantine campaign of the 1830s and early 1840s.

True to form, Louis ventured no such audacious conclusions. His account of the epidemic, published in 1839, was devoted to reporting the results of detailed clinical and postmortem examinations of the few fatal cases of yellow fever that occurred after he and his associates had reached Gibraltar near the end of the epidemic. Without a doubt, he concluded, the epidemic disease in Gibraltar was a specific entity, namely, yellow fever. It was also Louis who, eleven years after the event, placed in summary numerical form the morbidity and mortality experience of those victims of the epidemic who had been seen by the French commissioners.

But Louis also pointed out that these many facts, whether pathological or statistical, did not answer the question of how yellow fever is transmitted. Neither contagion nor noncontagion had been proved (or, unfortunately, disproved). Nor could the importation/nonimportation issue be resolved. Reasoning with the analogy of smallpox, a familiar model of contagious disease, Louis saw indications that yellow fever, too, might be contagious.[30] Smallpox was known to present itself "sporadically," that is, at times and in places where no epidemic was manifest. Yellow fever, it was said, also sometimes appeared sporadically and therefore could be usefully compared with this truly contagious disease. An atmospheric in-

---

between 1821 and 1867," pp. 572–575) has described the many participants in, especially, the noncontagionist campaign. The foremost spokesman of contagionism remained wholly unpersuaded. William Pym chaired the review board of the British army that had looked into the Gibraltar epidemic, a board which decided, by a vote of five to two, that yellow fever was a contagious disease. Pym's arguments included the specificity of yellow fever and the fact that it attacks a victim but once, both elements in the smallpox analogy. From this contagionist conclusion there was drawn the further conclusion that yellow fever was an importable disease and was not caused by changed local conditions. Pym, an acerbic figure slightly, if at all, less impassioned by his convictions than was Chervin by his, shared his views with a wider public in *Observations upon Bulam, Vomito-Negro or Yellow Fever, with a Review of 'A Report upon the Diseases of the African Coast by Sir William Burnett and Dr. Bryson,' Proving its Highly Contagious Powers* (London: John Churchill, 1848); extracts from the army board's deliberations appear on pp. 298–311.

30. On the smallpox analogy, see Margaret Pelling, *Cholera, Fever and English Medicine, 1825–1865* (Oxford: Oxford University Press, 1978), pp. 248–253.

fluence, in contrast, could be expected to affect many persons within a brief period of time. Still, sporadic appearance was dangerously ambiguous. Yellow fever could arise, and perhaps had arisen at Gibraltar, "independently of anything coming from America." This strongly suggested noncontagion. Louis observed, however, that such a conclusion need "not follow" from the data presented. The facts, he admitted, just do not permit one to state that "yellow fever is not contagious." But neither did they allow one to conclude that yellow fever is contagious.[31]

Louis had no solution to the old dilemma, and he knew it. His inconclusive speculations commanded but two in a work of almost four hundred pages. He offered, furthermore, no comment at all on the policy implications of the commissioners' inquiries. Trousseau did no more and was equally perplexed. It was, in fact, thirty years before he publicly discussed the matter. Speaking before the Academy of Medicine in 1857, he still found need to question Chervin's ready solution to the problem. His lamented colleague, he observed, now dead some fifteen years, had pretended to find in Gibraltar truly ripe "paludic conditions," those damp marshlike conditions held to be favorable to the production of a morbific miasma. But Gibraltar, Trousseau observed to no one's surprise, was merely a "rock" and in the summer of 1828 it was, as usual, a dry and well-drained rock.[32]

Chervin had held that the paludic or marsh fevers and yellow fever were really variations upon a single disease, yellow fever probably representing its most advanced and thus most severe condition. This was a crucial matter, for, as already has been emphasized, the specificity of yellow fever was the essential foundation for the further development of the epidemiology of the disease. In Chervin's system, insistence upon the nonspecificity of disease, and his belief that lesser fevers might evolve to become dangerous illnesses such as yellow fever, moved hand-in-hand with the nonimportationist outlook.[33] Trousseau, however, like Louis, categorically denied the notion of evolving disease entities and accepted yellow fever as an independent and stable clinical entity.

But Trousseau might disagree with Chervin and still have no solution. In 1857 his thoughts tended toward the contagionist explanation of Gibraltar's misfortune. He did not, however, insist upon this conclusion and phrased it in the conditional. Unable to specify suitable local causes, he

31. Louis, *Researches on the Yellow Fever of Gibraltar*, pp. 373–374.

32. Trousseau, in ["Discussion"] "Rapports. *Mémoire sur la fièvre jaune*, par M. le docteur Dutroulau, etc.," *Bulletin de l'Académie impériale de médecine* 22 (1856–1857): 1203.

33. Chervin, *De l'identité de nature des fièvres d'origine paludéene de différens types, à l'occasion de deux mémoires de M. Rufz, sur la fièvre qui a régné à la Martinique de 1836 à 1841; et de l'urgence d'abolir les quarantines relatives à cette maladie* [Rapport fait à l'Académie royale de médecine] (Paris: J. B. Baillière, 1842), pp. 65–78, 93–96.

was tempted to consider imported causes, but, in his discussion (which was conducted a full generation after the event) he attempted no close analysis and cited no telling old or new facts. Like Louis, Trousseau did not discuss the quarantine issue.

The publications of the three French commissioners, like those of British and other French observers of the Gibraltar epidemic, led to neither settled epidemiological or etiological conclusions nor agreed-upon administrative measures. While much testimony had been gathered, that evidence did not permit the definitive resolution of even one of the important outstanding questions. Within the British medical community, the contentions voiced early in the century by the contagionists Colin Chisholm and Gilbert Blane and by their many noncontagionist opponents were renewed by the epidemic of 1828. A clearer resolution of the issues was not found across the Channel than had been provided by the French commissioners.[34] Later observers faced these disputes with growing impatience. They admitted that assertiveness might support confidence, but realized that it offered no assurance of the validity of either principles or conclusions. Etienne Rufz de Lavison was a physician who had had extensive experience with yellow fever in the French Antilles, and he showed himself to be one of the most judicious minds to follow the unending dispute over the nature and spread of the disease. He wrote, in 1857:

34. In addition to William Pym's many battles, the principal exchange involved David Barry and Hugh Fraser. Their publications are: (1) [J. Johnson] "Gibraltar Fever" [Report on Barry's paper before the Royal College of Physicians], *Medico-Chirurgical Review*, n.s., 12 (1830): 539–540; (2) Fraser, "Review of the Facts and Arguments brought forward by Dr. Barry, at the Royal College of Physicians, Relative to the late Epidemic Fever in the Fortress of Gibraltar," ibid., 13 (1830): 337–350; (3) Barry, "Remarks on the Gibraltar Fever," *London Medical and Physical Journal*, n.s., 9 (1830): 379–397; (4) Fraser, "Letter from Mr. Hugh Fraser, late Surgeon to the Civil Hospital of Gibraltar," ibid., 10 (1831): 31–33; (5) Barry, "On the Gibraltar Epidemic of 1828," ibid., 10 (1831): 92–98 — this is Barry's paper read to the Royal College of Physicians and in effect a summary statement of his experience working with the French commission in Gibraltar; (6) Fraser, "Reply to Dr. Barry's Remarks on the Gibraltar Epidemic of 1828," ibid., 10 (1831): 202–224, 304–318, 399–413; (7) Barry, "Remarks on the Gibraltar Epidemic," ibid., 10 (1831): 475–494, 11 (1831): 1–23, 96–107; (8) [J. Johnson] "Remarks on the Gibraltar Epidemic," *Medico-Chirurgical Review*, n.s., 14 (1831): 69–80. The papers published in the *London Medical and Physical Journal* received occasional comment by the editor. It was, apparently, the medical reaction to the Philadelphia yellow-fever epidemic of 1793 that launched the noncontagionist program (Ackerknecht, citing La Roche, "Anticontagionism between 1821 and 1867," pp. 570–571), but some British physicians and surgeons were at the same time also asserting a contagionist interpretation of yellow fever. Their stand was announced by Colin Chisholm (*An Essay on the Malignant Pestilential Fever introduced into the West Indian Islands from Boullam, on the coast of Guinea, as it appeared in 1793 and 1794* [London: Dilly, 1795]) and continued by Blane and Pym. Fraser, a noncontagionist, and Barry, something of a contagionist, sustained the dispute with new evidence and old arguments.

What is the origin of epidemics? Do they result from the development of slight cases [that is, evolve from a local and less serious miasmatic disease] or are they brought in from outside? Science has not closed the book on this matter. What we need are numerous and rigorous investigations, conducted with the assistance of public authorities. We have a model for this in the investigation in which M. Trousseau took part [that is, the Gibraltar commission]. Unfortunately, these gentleman have given us only raw materials and we are still waiting [after 30 years!] for the message which these materials might provide. We need a great many investigations of this kind. Until we have them, it is more prudent to doubt all the facts that have been put before us.[35]

The Character of the Investigation

Rufz's words reflect two generations of disappointment and deception. They turn attention from the simplistic etiological conclusions and doctrinal confusion of the 1830s and 1840s and direct it upon what was increasingly seen to be the first necessity in the analysis of an epidemic. One must attend to the basic question of which epidemiological facts are relevant and to the problem of how such facts are to be collected and marshalled so as to produce a reliable message. A methodological program, but one not readily articulated, was inherent in these demands. Rufz's appeal was launched only four years before yellow fever struck Saint-Nazaire. Since Trousseau took an active part in the 1857 discussions at the Academy of Medicine, Rufz's critical words could not fail to remind academicians, including François Mélier, of the problems associated with the conduct of the earlier inquiry.

Of these problems the most important was the late arrival of the commissioners in Gibraltar. They were by no means the first observers on the scene of the epidemic. British and Spanish physicians followed events from the outset, but they concentrated on combating the disease and only secondarily studied it closely. The charge to the French was to analyze an epidemic, not practice medicine. Louis, a decade later, expressed regret for the delayed arrival, stressing that when an epidemic strikes one must seize the occasion. Ordinary diseases, he observed, can be studied on any ordinary day but

> it is not so with an epidemic. The description of it must remain as it was made at the time of its prevalence. We can add nothing to it, we can take nothing from it; we cannot assure ourselves by [subsequent] observation, of

35. Rufz de Lavison, in ["Discussion"] "Rapports. *Mémoire sur la fièvre jaune*, par M. le docteur Dutroulau, etc.," *Bulletin de l'Académie impériale de médecine* 22 (1856–1857): 1214. Chervin thought little of Rufz's interpretations; see his critical account of the latter's study of epidemic yellow fever in the Antilles, above, note 33.

the fidelity and ability of its observers. Two epidemics of the same disease differ more or less from each other. How very important, then, becomes the careful observation of an epidemic![36]

But the commissioners, as has been seen, did not really observe their epidemic. They observed instead its tame concluding weeks. (Louis's scalpel opened only some two dozen of the last seventy-six victims, that is, those seen by the French commissioners.) Their main preoccupation was to assemble recollections and opinions stated by others regarding the earlier stages of the outbreak. Hence, the *Documens* in no way met Louis's standard of description, that it be made at the very moment of an epidemic's prevalence.

A delay of this kind poses a lesser problem for the noncontagionist. A miasmatic influence may be expected to linger for a longer or a shorter period in a locality, and the matter of the precise time of appearance of the first victim, while surely of interest, would not command a decisive position in the analysis. It seemed, however, that persons wishing to examine the possibility of the nonlocal origin of a disease faced a serious obstacle if they were absent when cases first became apparent. The "contact," whether inanimate or animate, would best be recognized at an early moment, preferably very near the time of contact. With diseases conveyed by ship, the moment of contact might be very brief indeed. Even with his rudimentary understanding of the disease, the nineteenth-century physician knew that the incubation period and the acute phase of yellow fever might in some instances be accomplished in less than two weeks. With the severe case, disease recognition might be certain and convalescence prolonged; the late-arriving observer could perhaps derive useful information under such circumstances. The less severe and the numerous subacute cases usually recovered quickly; they then disappeared from the public and medical eye, had they been recognized at all.

In addition to these problems, medical surveillance of ports was lax. European physicians were unfamiliar with the disease. Yellow fever could be confused with other diseases and escape detection. With each passing day an informed sanitary officer or an alert physician interested in the possibility of either importation or contagion was further removed from the information that he most needed, namely, an exhaustive account of the conditions surrounding the appearance of the earliest victim or victims.

An investigator who had collected testimony that could not be corroborated, or who studied the case of a victim whose situation presented no demonstrable connections, might still attempt to imagine a set of presump-

36. Louis, *Researches on the Yellow Fever of Gibraltar*, p. xix.

tive linkages between specific conditions and the appearance of a specific case of yellow fever. In Gibraltar there was occasion for little more than this. Here there was slight hope for securing a closed chain of connections that might confirm the importationist hypothesis, render the contagionist position more compelling, or definitively disprove either or both. The non-contagionist did not need this kind of evidence and in general did not regard human sickness as one of the conditions of the sickness of others.

Nonetheless, the noncontagionist might have reason to undertake case-tracing in a serious manner, regardless of how the first case was handled. Chervin did not, but Mélier and Buchanan did. These later epidemiologists had learned that the presence or absence of connections between cases provided a fundamental datum of their science and that a field investigation was to be directed toward obtaining reliable information on just this point. The movement of a disease through a population was the proper subject of the science. During the course of an epidemic investigators would need to hold in abeyance traditional conclusions such as contagion and noncontagion until reaching solid grounds for reasoning on those conclusions. The new information might confirm an old conclusion or it might reject it, but the process of gathering that information was, it had become clear, a task that was not to be constrained by the demands of one or another entrenched theoretical position. Nothing was easy in this program (one does not simply walk away from often unacknowledged preconceptions), yet the program itself announced the arrival in the study of epidemics of a new open-mindedness, a strong phenomenological bias. This bias might only encourage the mere collection of facts and avoidance of conclusions, yet it could also stimulate more direct and creative reasoning on the accumulated data, reasoning now freed from the ready dicta of the contagionist or noncontagionist camp.

A second parameter closely associated with timing and, indeed, dependent upon it, is the character of the inquiry, the kind of inquiry that an investigator finds it possible to conduct. The French commissioners in Gibraltar had no choice but to gather their information well after the event. Often apparent fact was nothing but opinion or uncertain memory. Worst of all, there was no way that these usually incomplete and often contradictory reports could be compared with either the scene of the events themselves or with written records kept during the epidemic. Many needed facts could not be established, contradictions could not be resolved, and testimony could not be verified.

These difficulties affected most seriously, again, the partisans of importation. The *Dygden* and the *Méta*, their masters and their crews, had long since disappeared. It was quite impossible to gather reliable information regarding the disease conditions that had prevailed aboard these ships during their transatlantic passage or about their health status upon arrival at Gibraltar. The same impossibility applied to the numerous other ships that reached Gibraltar from the Americas in the summer of 1828, whose arrivals received no notice at all.

One consequence of this unfortunate situation was that reports on yellow-fever epidemics often resembled nothing so much as a scorecard. The medical profession was polled and truth was established by a vote. Chervin was a leader in this practice. In his unpublished documents brought from America, this consummate epidemiological gamesman assembled medical opinion to show that, among experienced New World physicians, 483 doctors voted yellow fever to be noncontagious and only 48 contagious, a comfortable 10:1 margin in informed opinion.[37] Mélier and Buchanan conducted no polls. Instead, they examined the movement of the disease through discrete populations. They were able to trace all (serious) cases and establish connections between each of these cases and also between each victim and presumed causal agencies. Their procedure and its success required that they be present during what Louis had called the prevalence of the epidemic, and they were; the French commissioners of 1828 were not.

A further parameter of the investigation of epidemic yellow fever deserves notice. It was agreed that severe cases of yellow fever constitute a distinct clinical entity; even Chervin had admitted this. The following several questions remained to be answered. Was yellow fever an obvious disease, easily identified before a background of other severe fevers? Was the disease setting within which yellow fever appeared itself distinctive? What, in fact, was to be understood by such a setting? How did or should one characterize the disease situation of a given place and time?

A comparison that offers more than mere analogical force illuminates these questions. During the nineteenth century the physician came increasingly to view illness as a disturbance of normal bodily or mental function. The concept of disease gradually lost its ontological status.[38] Illness, like health, was not a definite and autonomous category of existence; a supposed entity, disease, did not come from without and impose itself upon

37. Dubois d'Amiens, "Notice historique sur M. Chervin," pp. xliv–xlv. One author was little persuaded by this form of argument. Decisions regarding the contagious or noncontagious nature of a disease, the anonymous writer observed, are not to be made "by collecting the mere opinions of physicians, however able, and counting them like the suffrages of electors, but by observing the circumstances under which the disease is propagated, and especially under which it seems to spread from sickly locations to remote and healthy districts." Anon., "Art. I.1. Minutes of Evidence before a Commission, etc.," *Edinburgh Medical and Surgical Journal* 35 (1831): 382.

38. See Owsei Temkin, "Health and Disease," in *The Double Face of Janus and Other*

a theretofore innocent recipient. Rather, disease, like health, represented a point or set of points along a continuum that runs from life, its forces intact, to death. One man's pleasure is another man's poison, and the body or mind responds accordingly.

Specific diseases do indeed exist and, although their specificity is reflected in a commonality of described symptoms and pathological findings, the individual is rare who exhibits these features in a supposedly typical mode. Each victim presents his or her affliction in his or her own way, within the general parameters of the disease in question. It is precisely the individualization of disease (and, to be sure, what each person deems health) that poses the fundamental task of the medical practitioner. The clinician, who is by schooling well apprized of the general, must constantly address the particular. He must cope with disease in an individual whose own "normal" is surely not the same as, yet is similar to, that of others; and he must approach that person's "pathology" or "abnormal" within the same constraints. Working on an individual level, the physician simply cannot attempt to comprehend aberrant functions — disease or some other impairment of function — without also attempting to formulate a reasonably precise notion of what unimpaired or normal activity for that individual might be or have been. Wide-ranging clinical experience is highly valued for precisely this reason. The sound judgement of an accomplished physician permits detection of often subtle changes that indicate a shift away from the patient's normal condition and the onset of what could become life-threatening alterations.

Just as the observer of the sick individual had need to discover, or devise, criteria for estimating the normal in order to grasp the dimensions of the abnormal, so the student of population phenomena needed comparable procedures and standards. Over the past several generations we have come to expect a numerical measure — crude death rate, infant mortality, morbidity, or any of numerous other indices — of social and public health norms. Population phenomena and number seem inseparable. Such thoughts and expectations were certainly present in the middle decades of the nineteenth century, yet the practical reality for both clinician and epidemiologist was far otherwise. It was in the 1830s, during the first flurry of regular empirical investigation and theoretical creation in the social sciences, that simple numerical procedures were introduced and tentatively employed. A primary provocation was the appalling condition of the labor-

---

Essays in the History of Medicine (Baltimore: Johns Hopkins University Press, 1977), pp. 419–440; Georges Canguilhem, *Le normal et le pathologique* (Paris: Presses Universitaires de France, 1966), pp. 69–95; M. D. Grmek, "La conception de la maladie et de la santé chez Claude Bernard," *Mélanges Alexandre Koyré*, 2 vols. (Paris: Hermann, 1964), 1:208–227.

ing classes in the new industrial cities; a second was the statesman's peren-
nial concern to have an exact measure of national power and potential.
Within this framework the whole domain of social statistics arose, which
at the outset dealt eclectically with population size and growth, economic
activity, literacy, religious affiliation, disease in its many forms, and much
else. Furthermore, the 1820s and 1830s also saw the emergence of efforts
to reason with these numbers. The principal contribution was made by
the Belgian astronomer, Adolphe Quetelet, who sought to discover the
mathematical laws he was confident lay hidden behind diverse social phenomena. Others used the new data to analyze the character of social structure and change and the relation of each to health and disease. This work
was closely related to, and sometimes indistinguishable from, early epidemiological investigation.[39]

The quantitative approach to hygiene and to health and disease was
at the outset descriptive and usually exceedingly simple, offering at most
an incomplete view of the phenomena of interest, and it long remained
so. Its quantitative content scarcely exceeded manipulation of sums and
differences. But another important if ill-defined intention was also present, namely, to use the mean (usually only an average) as a measure of
normality. Quetelet's celebrated conception of the average man, as well as
the very notion of the "normal" curve, reinforced this usage, however abu-
sively. This numerical approach, despite its appeal of being the method
best suited to exact science, was itself only a refined way to obtain a grasp
on the normal or nonaberrant condition of one or another social or disease condition.

Now epidemiology deals with both the social situation and the disease
condition. It is, in fact, the science of disease as the latter manifests itself
in a social setting. What has been added, in comparison with the clinician's view of disease, is a population and the many parameters that might
affect such a population. The physician wishes to understand how such

39. See Edwin Chadwick, *Report on the Sanitary Condition of the Labouring Population of Gt. Britain*, ed. M. W. Flinn (Edinburgh: Edinburgh University Press, 1965), pp. 1–
73; J. M. Eyler, *Victorian Social Medicine. The Ideas and Methods of William Farr* (Baltimore: Johns Hopkins University Press, 1979); A. F. La Berge, "Public Health in France and
the French Public Health Movement, 1815–1848" (Knoxville: Ph.D. diss., University of Tennessee, 1974); William Coleman, *Death Is a Social Disease. Public Health and Political Economy in Early Industrial France* (Madison: University of Wisconsin Press, 1982). Also M. J.
Cullen, *The Statistical Movement in Early Victorian Britain. The Foundations of Empirical
Social Research* (New York: Barnes and Noble, 1975); V. L. Hilts, *Statist and Statistician:
Three Studies in the History of Nineteenth-Century English Statistical Thought* (New York:
Arno Press, 1981); T. M. Porter, *The Rise of Statistical Thinking, 1820–1900* (Princeton:
Princeton University Press, 1986).

parameters pertain to his client; the epidemiologist will explore many of the same factors, but he seeks to relate them to the condition of the community. I have emphasized the quantitative aspect of the growing interest in social phenomena because, ultimately, social science and epidemiology came to view number as the basic index of any population process. But, and this is an essential qualification, although this thought was entertained throughout the nineteenth century, it was not until century's end that numerical analysis of such data began to transcend an elementary level and afford the epidemiologist truly powerful new tools.[40] Statistics, along with microbiology constituting the scientific core of modern epidemiology, is thus a late addition to epidemiology. In its absence numerical measures of normality were either infrequently ventured or subject to great and just reserve.

What, then, might an aspiring epidemiologist do when, lacking the rigor of a numerical statement, he attempted to apprehend the normal condition of a setting within which an epidemic occurred? He did what he had always done, and he did it either well or poorly. He sought to determine what had been the sanitary condition of the community when the epidemic had begun and how it had changed during the epidemic. His approach was purely qualitative and his method was description: description of diseases, if these were subject to direct inspection, and especially description of prevailing environmental conditions. The epidemiological "normal" at Gibraltar, for example, was not expressed (insofar as anyone attempted to describe it at all) in terms of mortality or natality, much less in terms of general morbidity or the incidence of particular diseases. Instead, brief verbal characterizations were offered, comprehensiveness was neither sought nor attained, no notion of standardization of description was considered, and, as might be expected, contradiction and confusion abounded. When Mélier visited Saint-Nazaire forty years later, he made no use of numerical measures of the vital condition of the town. But by drawing on the medical and other resources of the community, he did attempt to determine which diseases (if any) were present, and to ascertain the prevailing meteorological situation and behavior of affected persons and objects related to maritime activities. All of these parameters were quite properly assigned to the total environmental or ecological setting of the disease. Buchanan proceeded no differently in Swansea.

Just what could, in fact, be said regarding the sanitary condition of Gibraltar when yellow fever struck? What was the "normal" situation on

40. See Hilts, *Statist and Statistician*, pp. 479–502, 547–576; D. A. MacKenzie, *Statistics in Britain, 1865–1930. The Social Construction of Scientific Knowledge* (Edinburgh: Edinburgh University Press, 1981), pp. 56–72 and passim.

the peninsula in the summer of 1828? Two things were obvious: various illnesses were present but not, apparently, uncommonly so; and yellow fever seemed to be a sudden arrival, one dramatically cast upon the town. Beyond this there was little agreement. Indeed, a chaos of opinion expressed itself. There was no common pattern to the many reports, and the French commissioners' own contribution, the *Documens*, provided no summary assessment of the matter. Jean Louis Geneviève Guyon, for example, a French observer not connected with the commission, thought that Gibraltar was a remarkably clean town, especially when compared to the filthy desolation he claimed to find in nearby Spanish towns and villages. Chervin, however, announced repeatedly that Gibraltar in general, and especially the most seriously afflicted districts within the town, were veritable cesspools in which miasmatic influences found ideal conditions for development.[41]

Strictly construed, sanitary condition referred to local environmental conditions, to temperature extremes, humidity, street filth, poor disposal of human and animal wastes, and unhygienic housing. Chervin and others paid little attention to that other sanitary condition, the prevailing burden of disease in the town on the eve and after the onset of yellow fever. It was agreed, however, that the disease situation in Gibraltar had not been unusual, whatever this might mean. When, forty years later, Mélier and Buchanan ascertained the local incidence of disease, they were deliberately seeking a standard for judging the central issue of whether yellow fever was in fact new or unusual, whether it was a genuine importation. In the absence of a prominent local fever, and given the sudden appearance of a serious fever known to be common in another land with which a specific transportation link could be demonstrated, it seemed unlikely that the new fever was only a changed and intensified form of some indigenous affliction. Certainly it was not the most economical explanation of that appearance. The argument depended upon possession of a reasonably sure baseline, a notion of the normal condition of local sanitary affairs. The important dialectic between the normal and the pathological thus reaches well beyond the familiar discourse of the clinical observer

41. Guyon, "Reflexions sur l'origine de la maladie de Gibraltar en 1828," *Journal complémentaire du Dictionnaire des sciences médicales* 37 (1830): 305–307; [Chervin], "Lettre sur l'épidémie de fièvre jaune . . . adressée par M. le docteur Chervin, à M. le docteur Monfalcon," pp. 66–68; Chervin, *De l'origine locale et de la non-contagion de la fièvre jaune qui a régné à Gibraltar en 1828, ou Réponse à quelques assertions émises par M. Guyon, dans la vue d'établir que cette maladie eut une origine exotique* (Paris: Imprimerie royale, 1832); Barry, "On the Gibraltar Epidemic of 1828," *London Medical and Physical Journal* 10 (1831): 92–98.

and medical practitioner; it is equally essential to the conceptualization of a public health inquiry and the interventions of preventive medicine.

In the realm of disease theory, the Gibraltar epidemic served to refine, support, and make notorious the major contentions of the noncontagionist view of yellow fever. To be sure, contagionists did not disappear after 1830, but their task was now seen to be very difficult. A contagionist had to prove the impossible. John Hennen, an eclectic theorist who knew the Mediterranean epidemic situation very well and who himself fell victim to the Gibraltar epidemic, wrote that "nothing can be more difficult to ascertain than the introduction of an invisible contagion; from the very nature of things, the proof is inferential."[42] Hennen wondered who but a special pleader, or a contagionist, could see the invisible, even with the mind's eye? The contagionist ignored the fact that personal contact, the crucial event in his interpretation, repeatedly failed to communicate the disease to susceptible persons. Still, this interesting fact was balanced by another fact, one dear to the contagionist. Overlooked or otherwise explained away by the noncontagionist was the sudden appearance of the disease after the arrival, usually by ship, of a demonstrably ill individual. Surely something had been imported, and surely that something was intimately connected with the human frame. But what, precisely, was it? Hennen was certainly right. Contagionists did argue that an "invisible contagion" had been introduced. Yet this very invisibility seemed to many merely a sign of insubstantiality. Contagionism defied the senses.

What would later become clear, largely through study of the Saint-Nazaire and Swansea epidemics, was the fact that importation was not limited to the sick human being, in whose body the contagionist saw the causal agent of disease. Miasmata, too, might travel long distances, especially when closed in small sailing ships, and upon arrival they could cause disease in a virgin port. Miasmata were the theoretical constructs of the noncontagionist, yet the latter could now also accept importation and reject local origins. Mélier and Buchanan knew nothing of the intimate nature of yellow fever's causal miasma and they entertained no suspicion at all that an intermediate host played a role in the transmission of yellow fever to man. They had learned, however, how to track an epidemic and how to use the details thus discovered to develop and defend a new view of the epidemic character of the disease.

42. Hennen, *Medical Topography of the Mediterranean*, p. 108.

II

Yellow Fever in the North

3

Saint-Nazaire: The Epidemic of 1861

On 4 August 1861, a sailor died of yellow fever at Indret, a naval station near the French port of Nantes. The following day another death occurred, now at Saint-Nazaire, some thirty miles west of Nantes. During the next several weeks over forty persons fell seriously ill, and two-thirds of them died; all were victims of yellow fever. The disease was not entirely unknown in the region, an isolated case (or cases) occasionally arriving aboard an inbound ship from America. The events at Saint-Nazaire, however, presented a new phenomenon, for this time an extensive epidemic had broken out among the local population.

Whatever the initial uncertainty or hesitation, observers at Saint-Nazaire soon acknowledged the appearance in their community of an unusual and unusually threatening disease. Few thought that this new fever was only the heightened form of a local fever. It was possible that the disease had been introduced from without, but in a manner as yet unknown. To convert this suspicion into a well-grounded demonstration required the rigorous evaluation of virtually everything that transpired during the course of the epidemic. Certain questions could not be avoided. By what means had the disease or its (unknown) causal agent been introduced? Could the precise time and place of introduction be specified? Could arrival of the disease be traced to the arrival of particular objects or persons?

Answers to these questions suggested a solution to the first general problem, how the disease had gained access to the community. This set the frame for further and equally important questions. Once imported, how did the disease move within the community? Were local environmental conditions relevant to that movement? What role, if any, did person-to-person communication play? Arriving in Saint-Nazaire while the epidemic was at its peak, François Mélier addressed these several questions. He launched an exhaustive inquiry into the hygienic conditions affecting the town and its residents, transient as well as permanent, and he and his associates were soon able to discover and trace all persons seriously afflicted by yellow fever. From this action followed all else. Transmission by personal contact was assayed and, with certain exceptions, denied; transmission by contact with ship's cargo or other goods (fomites in general) was also assayed and denied; however, transmission by connection with an infected ship, the nature of which required specification, was tested and affirmed.

The inexperience with yellow fever of the inhabitants of Saint-Nazaire was a boon to epidemiological inquiry. Immunity among older persons had doubtlessly been widespread at Gibraltar in 1828, although ascertaining how common it actually was proved impossible. Persons in Saint-Nazaire who were immune to yellow fever constituted a vanishingly small minority, composed of those few individuals connected with commerce and the navy who had contracted the disease in the Antilles or in Africa. Here then, as in Swansea a few years later, was a large susceptible population occupying a generally healthy site. These favorable circumstances —for disease but also for study—were not duplicated in regions where yellow fever was endemic or where it returned with some frequency, as it did in the Americas or on the Iberian peninsula.

The Investigator, the Epidemic, the Port

François Mélier (1798–1866) was sixty-three years old when epidemic yellow fever entered Saint-Nazaire. He grew up in southwestern France, near Limoges, and completed his medical training in Paris in 1823.[1] An astute clinician and active practitioner, he is credited with being among the earliest to perceive the advantage of surgical intervention in dealing with the risk of caecal perforation in acute appendicitis. By the 1830s, however, his interest in matters of public hygiene had begun to dominate, and would ultimately displace, his earlier medical concerns.

During the 1840s he published a series of remarkable essays in the broad domain of public health and related public policy. These were years when leadership in such matters still belonged to France, although English and other investigators were rapidly becoming serious rivals. Mélier came of age in the Paris of the founders of modern French public hygiene, Jean-Noël Hallé, Jean-Baptiste Parent-Duchâtelet, and Louis René Villermé. He shared with these men, and with the wide-ranging French public health movement, the view that scrupulous firsthand investigation is the *sine qua non* of any plan of action in the realm of public hygiene.[2]

1. Jules Bergeron, "Eloge de M. Mélier," *Mémoires de l'Académie nationale de médecine* 36 (1888): 1–30; François Mélier, *Candidature à l'Académie de médecine: Titres de M. Mélier* (Paris: 1841). Also William Coleman, "Medicine against Malthus: François Mélier on the Relation between Subsistence and Mortality," *Bulletin of the History of Medicine* 54 (1980): 23–42.

2. See A. F. La Berge, "Public Health in France and the French Public Health Movement, 1815–1848" (Knoxville: Ph.D. diss., University of Tennessee, 1974); E. H. Ackerknecht, "Hygiene in France, 1815–1848," *Bulletin of the History of Medicine* 22 (1948): 117–155; William

Mélier's study of how to avoid the health risks of employment in the coastal marshes where sea-salt was prepared, and his sharp rejection of the idea that work in the tobacco factory was harmless — this being a favorite notion of Parent-Duchâtelet — are classic works in the early history of occupational medicine.[3] After 1850, Mélier assumed a variety of positions with the sanitary services of the French government. In this role, he became deeply involved in the sanitary affairs of the city of Marseilles. The primary French port in regular connection with plague areas in the Levant, Marseilles continued to maintain a strong defensive posture. Long after the last major intrusions of the plague into the western Mediterranean (1720-1743), quarantine and the surveillance of infection-bearing objects (fomites) were still upheld in Marseilles. The city was the principal focus for serious discussion of quarantine measures in France. But Mélier recognized the necessarily international dimensions of these discussions, a realization that led him to convene, under the auspices of the Second Empire, the first International Sanitary Conference, held in Paris in 1851. For the remainder of his career, he continued to support these conferences and other approaches to international surveillance and control of communicable disease. Active till the end of his career, he served during the Crimean War as coordinator of sanitary services for the French army in Russia and then served again in Italy in 1860.

Obviously, Mélier arrived in Saint-Nazaire well prepared for the needs of the occasion. He had spent a lifetime studying crowd diseases and evaluating the conditions under which these diseases began, spread, and disappeared; he had accumulated abundant experience with the administrative procedures involved in conducting a public-health investigation. The sureness and clarity of his report on the Saint-Nazaire epidemic — his most distinguished as well as his final contribution to medicine and epidemiology — reveals his readiness and ability to deal with virtually all parameters of a sudden and utterly unexpected outbreak of one of the most confusing of diseases.[4]

Coleman, *Death Is a Social Disease. Public Health and Political Economy in Early Industrial France* (Madison: University of Wisconsin Press, 1982). Also J. M. Eyler, *Victorian Social Medicine. The Ideas and Methods of William Farr* (Baltimore: Johns Hopkins University Press, 1979).

3. François Mélier, "Rapport sur les marais salants," *Mémoires de l'Académie royale de médecine* 13 (1847): 611-706; "De la santé des ouvriers employés dans les manufactures de tabac," ibid., 12 (1846): 604-648.

4. Mélier, "Relation de la fièvre jaune survenue à Saint-Nazaire en 1861," *Mémoires de l'Académie impériale de médecine* 26 (1863): 1-223; also issued as an independent volume (Paris: J. B. Baillière, 1863). The work consists of three parts, to each of which are added extensive "Pièces justificatives." The former two constitute Mélier's own presentation of the facts of the epidemic and his discussion thereof; the latter reproduces the voluminous docu-

Mélier reached Saint-Nazaire on 11 August 1861 and found the epidemic still very much underway. It was M. Saillant, a mechanical engineer aboard the tug *Chastang*, who had died of an unusual and fulminating disease at Indret on 4 August. Charles François Eloy died the next day at Saint-Nazaire (see chapter 1). Like Saillant, Eloy was carried off by a singular and uncontrollable disease. That same day, the fifth of August, physicians and public officials in the two ports realized, quite independently, that each faced a potentially grave epidemic situation: three new cases had appeared at Indret and seven new cases had followed Eloy's at Saint-Nazaire.

With these alarming events began the Saint-Nazaire yellow-fever epidemic of 1861. By the end of the epidemic, the last new case appearing on 31 August and the final death on 5 September, a total of forty-one persons had fallen ill and twenty-eight had died. Cases or deaths occurred in Saint-Nazaire and in nearby villages; at Indret; at Lorient, approximately seventy-five miles by sea west of Saint-Nazaire; and, most astonishing of all, for days on end aboard the *Aréquipa* as she sailed across the Atlantic from the Breton port to Cayenne in French Guiana.

Few doubts arose regarding the identity of the disease. In Saint-Nazaire, and especially at the naval station at Indret, there were physicians who knew yellow fever well, having tended numerous cases at overseas stations. At Indret the outbreak was brief and limited in extent but nonetheless spectacular.[5] The entire crew of the *Chastang* contracted yellow fever and all five men died in very short order (within two to five days); the case fatality rate had reached 100 percent. August Raynaud, inspector of naval medical services, was summoned from Paris, reaching Indret probably on 7 August, and a thorough inquiry was begun into the immediate and remote circumstances of this localized outbreak.

No other cases of yellow fever manifested themselves, early or late, at Indret or elsewhere along the lower Loire Valley. The first four victims, struck down with extraordinary suddenness and violence, gave the attending physician no epidemiologically useful information. The final victim, Fouché, who visited his fellow sailors with the physician before he himself succumbed to yellow fever, did offer a telling suggestion. The *Chastang* and her barges while at Saint-Nazaire had delivered a set of new boilers to a naval transport ship, the *Cormoran*. The *Chastang* then left Saint-

---

mentary records of the epidemic (ship reports, case histories, physicians' accounts, etc.), a veritable archive of Saint-Nazaire's experience. To the independent publication were added the text of the discussion of Mélier's preliminary report to the Academy of Medicine, published also in the Academy's *Bulletin* [28 (1862–1863): 646–695, 834–891, 977–1039], and a French translation of the English quarantine law of 27 June 1825 (6 Geo. 4, c. 78).

    5. Mélier, "Relation de la fièvre jaune survenue à Saint-Nazaire," pp. 119–123.

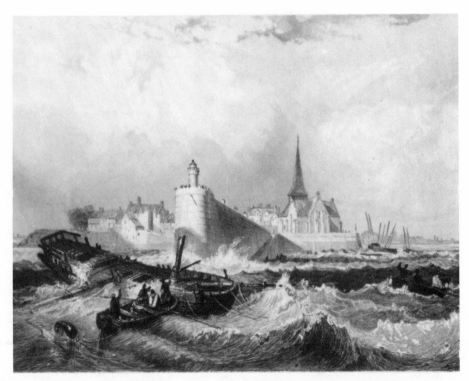

Saint-Nazaire before 1850. Shown are the Old Mole, offering some protection from open water to the south and west, and, to the right of the church, the landing stage that offered the town's only basis for maritime activity. Frequent or large shipping could not be received. (Courtesy of the Bibliothèque nationale.)

Nazaire on 29 August and reached Indret the same day. Fouché reported these events as follows:

> A ship from Havana, the *Anne-Marie* [see map location 1], was almost touching us; our stern [see map location 2] lay below her bowsprit. Throughout our stay (from 19 to 29 August) we maintained this position. This ship was loaded with sugar, packed in well-stowed boxes. Curiosity took us aboard, where we stayed only a brief moment (about fifteen minutes). While there we learned that during the crossing [from Cuba] two men had died and that the crew, upon arrival, had fled the ship, saying that they did not want to remain aboard their poisoned vessel one moment longer. These deserters were replaced by independent stevedores recruited in Saint-Nazaire.[6]

6. Ibid., p. 120.

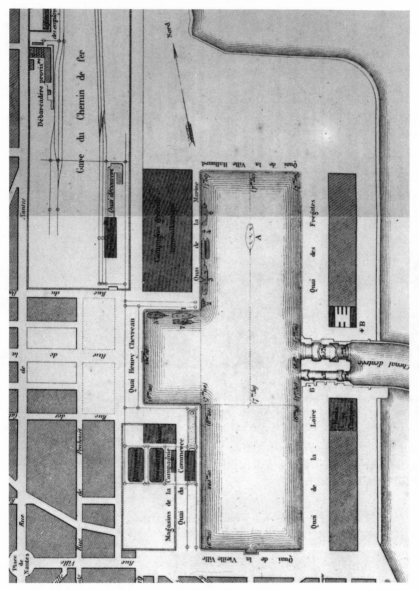

Port of Saint-Nazaire, 1861. The *Anne-Marie* stood first at location 1 and was later moved to location A. She was then sent across the Loire to Mindin. (*Mémoires de l'Académie impériale de médecine* 26 [1863]: Pl. 1.)

This information, collected on the afternoon of 4 August, became known in Saint-Nazaire only later in the investigation. Events at Indret were then reconciled with and found to confirm conclusions that observers in the port at the mouth of the Loire were already reaching.

After Eloy fell ill on the second of August, new cases of yellow fever at Saint-Nazaire followed rapidly. Five new victims appeared on the fifth and the last appeared on the thirty-first.[7] There was no question that most, but not all, of the cases were persons who had helped unload the *Anne-Marie*. Most had passed in and out of the ship's hold many times and others had remained there for an extended period. There were, however, a few cases that betrayed no obvious connection of any kind with the vessel. Informed of the course of these events, the Minister of Agriculture, Commerce, and Public Works — with whom responsibility for the sanitary surveillance of French ports then rested — dispatched his General Inspector of Sanitary Services, Mélier, to the stricken town.

Within a few days of his arrival (11 August), Mélier had concluded that the epidemic disease had been imported, probably aboard the *Anne-Marie*. He acted quickly, launching a sanitary program which, in looking to the future, demanded the introduction of revised and rigorously enforced procedures for ensuring the cleanliness of any suspect ship seeking entrance to the harbor; with an eye on the present, the program called for a concerted effort to locate every person suspected of having the disease. His objective was to collect exact and exhaustive information regarding the movement of those persons or of perhaps infected objects that had been in contact with or otherwise under the influence of the *Anne-Marie*.

In addition to the information received from Indret, Mélier requested and received from attending physicians in Saint-Nazaire detailed reports on the progress of each case of yellow fever in the town or nearby villages. These were combined with other reports on further extensions of the disease. The transport ship *Cormoran*, for example, was docked north of the *Anne-Marie* between 31 July and 6 August (see map location 6); she then moved somewhat closer and on 10 August sailed for Lorient. All six members of her crew had been healthy while in Saint-Nazaire and remained so until shortly after arrival at Lorient on the fourteenth. Two men then fell ill, one dying 19 August and the other 26 August. There could be absolutely no doubt that yellow fever was the cause of these deaths. One observer at Lorient was a naval physician who had just returned from Ha-

7. For Mélier's general narrative of events at Saint-Nazaire, upon which I draw for my own account on the next several pages, see ibid., pp. 16–35, and the relevant "Pièces justificatives."

vana, where epidemic yellow fever, the very "origin of our affair," Mélier would later remark, was then reigning.[8]

A fleet of steam ferries operated between Saint-Nazaire and Lorient. Occupying a dock position immediately west of the *Anne-Marie*, the ferry *Lorient No. 6* (see map location 5) stood at this quay between 28 and 30 July, and again between 2 August and the morning of 4 August. Upon reaching Lorient on the evening of the fourth, two members of the crew were reported ill. One, a stoker, died on the tenth and was not examined by a physician until the day before his death. The other, the cabin boy, at first thought his distress was due to an accidental fall during the passage. By the sixth, however, he was seriously ill and thereafter was closely observed and cared for by the health officer of the port. He began convalescence on the nineteenth and returned to complete health. From neither these victims, nor from those aboard the *Cormoran*, nor from the ship itself, did the disease spread to other persons, either while in passage or when in port at Lorient.

Between 2 and 5 August the brig *Dardanelles* was tied alongside and thus immediately south of the *Anne-Marie* (see map location 7). The *Dardanelles* had just returned from the Gulf of Guinea and the African coast. En route, and until 8 August, her crew, previously exposed to one of the most deadly climates a European could face, had all remained healthy. On the eighth, however, the cabin boy of the *Dardanelles* (who often crossed the deck of the *Anne-Marie*) fell seriously ill, no doubt with yellow fever. Only weeks later did he recover.

Seeking completeness, Mélier collected information regarding men and ships that did not appear to manifest yellow fever but that nonetheless had to be held under suspicion. The *Chastang* had towed two barges into the port of Saint-Nazaire and was docked with them near the *Anne-Marie* during the latter's first days of unloading. Five persons were aboard these barges but only one crewman boarded the *Anne-Marie*. None of these persons contracted "yellow fever strictly speaking" but all felt somewhat ill and physicians at Indret decided that their sickness did bear the peculiar cachet of yellow fever.[9] All had been in close contact with the dying men aboard the *Chastang*, caring for the ill and carrying the cadavers when death arrived. Nevertheless, none seemed to have contracted a genuine case of yellow fever or other serious disease from the moribund.

Of all the events associated with the epidemic at Saint-Nazaire none was more singular than the experience of the *Aréquipa*.[10] Information re-

8. Ibid., p. 21.
9. Ibid., p. 24. The distinctive features of this cachet were not discussed.
10. Ibid., pp. 25–27, 155–160.

garding this ship first became available months after the epidemic in Saint-Nazaire had ceased. The *Aréquipa* had reached Saint-Nazaire from Sierra Leone on 23 July. She came from another fearsome and unhealthy station, but all aboard were and had long been in excellent health. Having discharged her cargo, she prepared to depart for America. In so doing, she was placed alongside the *Anne-Marie* (see map location 7, prior to arrival of the *Dardanelles*). The *Aréquipa* remained in this location from 26 July to 1 August and then set sail. Her passage was delayed in the Bay of Biscay, but she then set a direct course for Cayenne. Five days out, the ship's second officer took violently ill; on the twelfth he died. Other cases of sickness followed. In all, eight crewmen were stricken and three died. The captain of the *Aréquipa* suspected yellow fever and acted accordingly, having the bodies and personal effects of the dead immediately cast into the sea and keeping a detailed account of sickness and death aboard his ship. Upon reaching Cayenne on 8 October, the *Aréquipa* was refused admission to the port. What could have been more bizarre? Here was a ship arriving directly from France in a port as foul and dangerous as any in the world, and the ship was immediately placed in quarantine because it threatened to import yellow fever from healthy northern climes into a tropical colony!

With the principal exception of the remarkable case of Alphonse Chaillon at Montoir (to be discussed in chapter 4), Mélier had now recorded all of the victims of yellow fever that had appeared in or in connection with Saint-Nazaire during the epidemic of August 1861. These were not simply the many cases that had been reported. Rather, an integral part of the inquiry had been to canvass the medical profession of the town and surrounding countryside, orally and by means of the telegraph, to ascertain the existence of all cases of serious disease of any kind. The few that were reported were investigated further; thus were located several of the stricken stevedores who had unloaded the *Anne-Marie* and who lived outside the town. The crew members who had left the ship were also traced and their condition established; none was in any way ill.

A fundamental problem with this investigation and with all early inquiries into epidemic yellow fever was the inability to identify subacute cases. Such cases can be expected to be relatively numerous, and they must be identified if one is to gain a fair sense of the incidence of the disease. But subacute cases were not sought out in Saint-Nazaire or elsewhere. Additionally, technical means for the required diagnosis were altogether unknown and remained so until the second third of the twentieth century. As a consequence, it is virtually certain that, in Saint-Nazaire and elsewhere, the number of persons sick with yellow fever was underreported, perhaps greatly so. Not only was the incidence of the disease thought falsely to be low, but the related case-fatality rate in these occasional epidemics was found to be very high. Perhaps the case-fatality rate was high, but this figure may have been only a function of placing the number of deaths (the numerator) over the number of very serious cases of sickness (the denominator), and not over the potentially larger number of all relevant cases of sickness.

The ability to trace in detail these several cases of serious illness was essential to the accomplishment of Mélier's task. The highly localized character of the epidemic, both in town and aboard ship, and the relatively small population involved (the *commune* of Saint-Nazaire in 1861 contained 6,500 inhabitants) meant that one could trace all cases — again, serious cases — with assurance.[11] Using this evidence, possible connections between cases or between particular victims and a possible source or sources of infection could be assessed. Real assurance in this realm had been quite impossible during the Gibraltar epidemic. As the vague story of the *Dygden* reveals all too well, a particularly weak point at Gibraltar had been the faulty knowledge, in fact the absence of knowledge, of the movement of ships into and within the port during the course of the epidemic. There was no problem on this score in the singular port and town of Saint-Nazaire.

The origins of Saint-Nazaire go back to neolithic times. For centuries Saint-Nazaire was only a minor fishing center, her small ships taking refuge from the open sea behind a narrow and rocky peninsula.[12] There was no port to speak of and no harbor for larger ships. International trade of large proportions passed nearby, but these ships were headed for the major port of Nantes, many miles up the Loire. Nantes was a leading French sugar refiner and her trade was especially intense with the Antilles.

Even in the eighteenth century there had been serious problems with navigation on the Loire. The river was shallow and shifting, constantly moving its main course and raising hazards to shipping. Much traffic to Nantes had to be transshipped to barges at the mouth of the river and then moved upstream to the port. These problems were only compounded by the new technology of the nineteenth century. The appearance of steam power, large iron ships, and the economy of scale increased the number of deep-draft vessels and gave promise of both speed and much-improved efficiency. The access of these ships to Nantes was severely limited, and

11. R. P. Kerviler, *Notice sur le port de Saint-Nazaire* (Paris: Imprimerie nationale, 1883), p. 72.

12. See Fernand Guériff, *Historique de Saint-Nazaire*, 2 vols. (Guérande: Imprimerie de "La Presqu'île," 1963), 1:194–221, 2:7–35; Kerviler, *Notice sur le port de Saint-Nazaire*, passim; Gaston Le Floc'h and Fernand Guériff, *Saint-Nazaire (Loire-Atlantique, 44)* (Colmar-Ingersheim: Editions S.A.E.P., 1974).

this fact assured the creation and dramatic development of Saint-Nazaire as a center of world trade.

After prolonged agitation, beginning under the First Empire, legislation was passed in 1845 authorizing construction of a new port for ocean-going ships at Saint-Nazaire. It proved necessary to create a harbor where not even rudiments existed. Massive stone walls were raised on the broad tidal flats flanking the Loire estuary. From these a narrow canal led to the sea. Locks placed in the canal assured access to the new harbor, itself a tidal basin. Opened on Christmas Day, 1856, the port of Saint-Nazaire provided twenty-six acres of protected water and ample quais atop the harbor walls. Railroad connections with Nantes and all of France were established in August 1857.

The new port could receive ships with a draft of some twenty feet and could thus handle tonnage well in excess of that which moved up the Loire. The success of Saint-Nazaire was breathtaking. In 1861, when yellow fever struck, 1,665 ships moved through the port; in 1856 neither a harbor nor international shipping had existed at Saint-Nazaire. The population of the town grew rapidly (1856: 5,424; 1865: 18,896; 1901: 35,813), but the city's economic life remained closely tied to the port.[13] Repeated efforts to create a broad industrial infrastructure met with only varied success. The port of Saint-Nazaire was subsequently greatly expanded, with new and connecting docks being built at Penhouët (1881) and elsewhere. The basin of 1856 remained essentially intact until the Second World War, when the German navy erected along its western perimeter a base for servicing submarines. This prodigious pile of concrete, the removal of which would undoubtedly entail enormous expenditure, persists today, replacing all the quais and water areas once associated with the *Anne-Marie*.

The original port and related installations had been constructed using government monies and loans and were well designed and constructed. Most of the new town, however, was a scene of speculative frenzy and urban chaos. One commentator, recalling the extravagances of the recent gold rush, called it our "little Breton California," jerry-built overnight, houses raised where streets were planned, a place to make money as fast as possible and move on.[14] In such a situation, sanitary measures received little consideration. Saint-Nazaire had no hospital until 1867, relying until then on the small *lazaretto* (with twelve beds and three nursing sisters) in Penhouët.

A mere four and one-half years after the opening of this new port, the

13. Kerviler, *Notice sur le port de Saint-Nazaire*, p. 203; Guériff, *Historique de Saint-Nazaire* 1:212.
14. Quoted in Guériff, *Historique de Saint-Nazaire* 2:9–10.

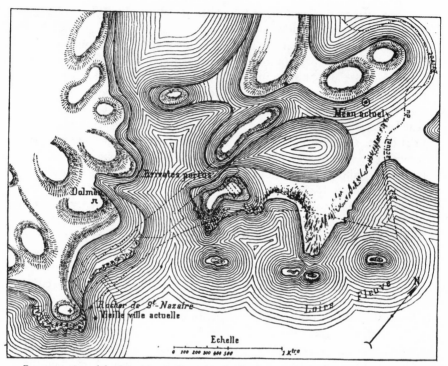

Reconstruction of the Saint-Nazaire littoral in the Gaulic period. The rectangular dotted lines indicate the areas on the tidal flats that were converted into the maritime port during the nineteenth century. The outer line traces the new shoreline. (Courtesy of the Bibliothèque nationale.)

Anne-Marie arrived. She carried an old product, sugar, as well as an old but unwelcome acquaintance, yellow fever. Remarkably enough, both came from a new trading partner, Cuba, whose sugar now moved freely into the French market and whose experience with yellow fever was notorious.

Saint-Nazaire, its boosters announced, was to become an essential link in the expansion of French foreign trade. The government obviously agreed, and assigned to Saint-Nazaire exclusive rights to carrying the post to Caribbean and Central American destinations. Saint-Nazaire was also the port of embarkation and sad return of the troops sent on the disastrous Mexican expeditions of 1861–1867.

The shock of the epidemic of 1861 was due not only to fear of yellow fever but to the fact that such a disease could enter Saint-Nazaire and do so in epidemic form. Her port facilities were well designed and soundly constructed. Her destiny, it was thought, was to lead France into an era of rapid industrial and mercantile expansion. But now the new town ap-

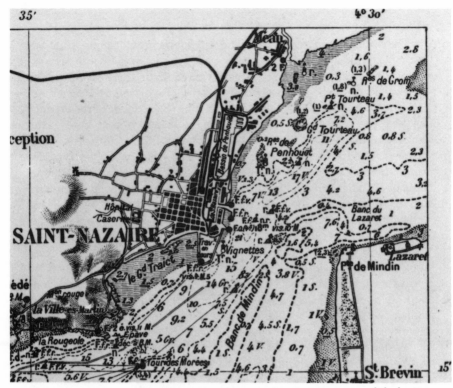

The mouth of the Loire ca. 1880. The two *bassins,* railroad connections, and the hygiene station at Mindin on the left bank of the river are shown, as is the rapid decrease in depth of the Loire. Depths in meters. (Courtesy of the Bibliothèque nationale.)

peared to succumb easily, as had so many older cities, to a fearsome pestilence. Such an assault would likely be followed by a serious decline in trade.

Happily, the epidemic of 1861 proved a limited affair. Yellow fever came, but yellow fever also went, and it never again returned to Saint-Nazaire in epidemic form. Confidence was quickly restored. And this was a good thing, for the volume of French foreign trade rose rapidly. Saint-Nazaire was a primary beneficiary of the abolition during the 1860s of duties on the importation of raw materials (including foodstuffs such as sugar) and of reduced tariffs on manufactured goods. This move toward free trade also opened foreign markets to French export goods.[15]

15. F. A. Haight, *A History of French Commercial Policies* (New York: Macmillan, 1931), pp. 30–42; M. S. Smith, *Tariff Reform in France, 1860–1900* (Ithaca: Cornell University Press, 1980), pp. 26–34.

An Epidemic at Sea: The *Anne-Marie*

The epidemic ashore and in neighboring ports provided important but incomplete evidence. If importation of yellow fever was a hypothesis worthy of consideration, a new set of facts was required. These facts included the experience of the *Anne-Marie*, for every case of yellow fever ashore appeared to implicate her in the epidemic. She formed part of the expanding fleet of vessels handling the Caribbean trade upon which Saint-Nazaire centered its interests. In 1861 alone, Mélier reported, the port received one hundred ships from the Americas, thirty-five of which had sailed from Havana.[16] Before the arrival of the *Anne-Marie* there had been no yellow fever at Saint-Nazaire, save the hypothetical occasional seaman who might have arrived ill but from whom the disease was neither known nor believed to have spread. Soon after the *Anne-Marie*'s arrival, cases of yellow fever sprang up in the town and along definite lines of physical connection.

Obvious questions thus had to be faced. Had there been yellow fever aboard the *Anne-Marie* in Havana or at sea? Did she carry yellow fever upon arrival in Saint-Nazaire? Forty years earlier, the French commissioners in Gibraltar, pondering the condition of the *Dygden*, had had to be content with rumor and fading recollections. Their ship had departed months earlier and they heard nothing from her captain. At Saint-Nazaire, the master of the *Anne-Marie*, Voisin, and the ship's records provided information of an entirely different character.

The *Anne-Marie* was a small wooden sailing ship of recent construction. She had sailed from Saint-Nazaire for Havana in March of 1861 and reached that port on 12 May. Malarial fevers were usually present in Havana and the town was well known for being a regular focus for other fevers, especially dengue fever and yellow fever. The disease situation in Havana in the early spring of 1861 had not been unusual or bad, but matters began to deteriorate rapidly in May. The French consul in the city then reported the simultaneous appearance of smallpox and yellow fever, the latter evolving into a particularly severe epidemic.[17]

The unhappy experience of Havana with yellow fever has been explained by the distinctive demographic and economic character of the city.[18] Urban yellow fever requires the presence of a virus, a mosquito, and a susceptible human being. In tropical and semitropical American cities the human situation was decisive for the continued presence of the disease. Cities

16. Mélier, "Relation de la fièvre jaune survenue à Saint-Nazaire," p. 5.
17. Ibid., citing a warning notice of 16 July 1861 sent to agents of the sanitary service by the Minister of the Navy and Colonies.
18. H. R. Carter, *Yellow Fever. An Epidemiological and Historical Study of Its Place of Origin* (Baltimore: Williams and Wilkins, 1931), pp. 17–21.

such as Rio de Janeiro, Guayaquil, Panama, and Havana were centers of economic activity and they possessed sizable European populations. Commerce radiated out from these cities; Rio de Janeiro and especially Havana were in frequent and direct contact with Europe. Each received from abroad a constant supply of yellow-fever susceptibles, including ships' crews. These cities also exercised a great attraction upon the population of their hinterlands, finding there another regular source of persons without immunity. Lastly, the birth rate in the American cities was high, and infants joined the susceptibles once they lost their short-lasting maternal immunity. Havana during the mosquito season was thus often a primary point for the spread of yellow fever.

After a month's stay in the Cuban capital, the *Anne-Marie* set sail for France. Her return was troubled by both weather and disease.[19] According to Captain Voisin, the crew upon departure (on 13 June) was generally healthy. Nonetheless, his men seemed fatigued and some reported feeling nauseated. A Havana physician advised the administration of purgatives; fourteen of the sixteen men aboard were duly purged. The voyage was much delayed by storms in the Straits of Florida: rain was heavy, long calms followed high winds, and the temperature was high. Once on the open sea, however, the ship's advance returned to normal and health remained good. Serious troubles then began on the morning of 1 July. A young man, previously in excellent condition, displayed bloodshot eyes, facial pallor, and shivering. By the time he had been undressed and put to bed he had become delirious. He never regained reason before dying on 5 July; the course of his fatal affliction had lasted some one hundred hours. A second crewman was also struck on the first and he, too, died on the fifth.

Aboard French merchant-ships with small crews, the captain acted as ship's physician, taking guidance from printed instructions provided by the Naval Ministry. Voisin tended to his ailing crewmen, using baths and lotions and — when the situation grew desperate — quinine, a remedy that offered no satisfaction. He also kept a detailed if nonprofessional record of symptoms, therapy, and resolution. Beginning on 2 July and continuing until the eighth, seven additional cases occurred. The last person to take ill was Voisin himself, his being no minor attack. None of these latter victims died, but convalescence for all was long.

The *Anne-Marie* was not merely a diseased ship; there had been a serious epidemic on board while crossing the Atlantic. Nine crewmen had fallen ill and two had died (a case-fatality rate of 22 percent). But had her crew suffered from yellow fever and then brought it to the shores of France?

19. Events aboard the *Anne-Marie* are described in Mélier, "Relation de la fièvre jaune survenue à Saint-Nazaire," pp. 6–11.

Captain and crew thought not—or spoke not. Voisin did not attempt to identify the disease (he gave it no name in his report but seemed to regard it as being a dry colic) and noted that only the two men who had not been purged had died. Mélier viewed the affair quite differently. "Ships' commanders," he observed, "do not in general admit [to having had] yellow fever [on board]. The captain of the *Anne-Marie* ascribed everything that he and his crew had suffered to excessive heat, storms, and fatigue. He was not beyond blaming even a comet that had passed by at the time. His own report of the matter, however, evokes quite a different idea; we cannot refuse to recognize here the presence of yellow fever."[20]

Upon arrival at Saint-Nazaire on 25 July, the *Anne-Marie*'s condition was anything but clean. Seven of her crew, including the captain, were still convalescing from an obviously serious attack of disease. Now, however, Nicolas Chervin's earlier triumph worked its untoward effect. Revision or suspension of quarantine rules and indifference to their enforcement had become common in France. French sanitary procedures after 1850 permitted authorities on the Mediterranean coast, who traditionally favored the idea of strong protective measures, to detain suspicious ships arriving from "yellow fever ports" for seven to ten days' observation.[21] On the Atlantic coast, however, where the climate was cooler and the voyage of an arriving ship much longer, the risks were thought to be smaller. Here ships from Havana, Cayenne, Dakar, or elsewhere within the usual reach of oceanic trade were to be allowed to move directly to an open quai if, during the last ten days of the voyage, neither death had occurred nor new cases of sickness had appeared on board. The two crewmen aboard the *Anne-Marie* had died on 5 July, twenty days before arrival; Voisin had fallen ill on the eighth, thirteen days before arrival. On reaching Saint-Nazaire the *Anne-Marie*, as Mélier soon was bitterly to observe, thus stood *"strictly within the letter of the law,"* and she was admitted.[22] She moved immediately to the Quai Jégou, and her captain and crew disembarked. Unloading was completed by 3 August. Only on the previous day, when Eloy, the ship's second officer, fell ill, did the first and still-vague suspicions surface that this ship, and these sanitary regulations, might pose a hazard to the port and perhaps to France at large.

Confident Diagnosis

Such a risk was great because, most observers agreed, a novel disease had reached France and that disease was none other than yellow fever.

20. Ibid., p. 9; Voison's report, ibid., pp. 117–119.
21. Ibid., p. 9.
22. Ibid.

Confusion with other fevers did not occur at Saint-Nazaire. Physicians —
especially naval physicians who had observed the disease in the Antilles,
Guiana, or Africa — recognized the clinical features and appreciated, too,
that the epidemiology of the disease offered further, important diagnostic
and prophylactic indications. Relying upon such expert witness, Mélier
approached the question with assurance. Unless, he sarcastically observed,
one cared to join those hopeless skeptics, whose penchant for system led
them to "contest everything and to deny the reality of movement even
while walking," the first fact of Saint-Nazaire was the presence of yellow
fever.[23]

This was a bold claim, given its author's total lack of experience with
the disease before meeting it in Saint-Nazaire. A Parisian physician did
not encounter yellow fever in his practice. But in the Breton port Mélier
examined a number of cases and, more important, insistently solicited
from attending physicians a detailed account of each case. These reports
constitute a remarkable series of case histories, each presented in full in
the *Pièces justificatives* attached to Mélier's general report on the epidemic.
The diagnosis of these cases was based principally upon symptoms. Physicians noted especially the severe headache that marked the onset of illness, the profound pain in the limbs and back that followed, in several
cases the progressive jaundice that became most marked near and after
death, occasional hemorrhage in the late stages of serious cases, and the
appearance of black vomit and stool.

Nineteenth-century French medicine is justly celebrated for its contributions to methods of diagnosis. These involved clinical description and
a systematic effort to correlate signs and symptoms with pathological findings disclosed by postmortem dissection. This latter correlation was virtually the emblem of the Paris school of medicine, yet it is disconcerting
to find that even in the 1860s it had not yet become a routine part of official medical investigation. The epidemic on the Loire posed a serious public threat. Twenty-eight persons died at Saint-Nazaire, yet only one postmortem examination was made.[24] Yellow fever was known to follow an
often varied course, and perhaps few observers expected to meet consistent pathological findings. Nonetheless, Pierre Charles Alexandre Louis
(in Gibraltar) had been far more attentive to this aspect of diagnosis than
were the several local, naval, and governmental physicians at Saint-Nazaire
and in nearby ports a third of a century later.

In any case, an additional set of diagnostic criteria was being brought
up in discussions of epidemic yellow fever — a set that moved beyond sign,

23. Ibid., p. 68.
24. Ibid., pp. 149–150.

symptom, and lesion to consideration of the ecology of the disease. Auguste Frédéric Dutroulau was a leading naval physician, experienced observer of yellow fever in Martinique and Guadaloupe, and author of a standard work on tropical (naval) medicine. He vigorously opposed Chervin's claims that yellow fever and paludal (that is, malarial) fevers were confined to marshy districts, shared a common origin, and were to be regarded as a single disease entity.[25] This notion, Dutroulau believed, was not only erroneous but posed a public danger. Paludal fevers were concentrated in marshy districts. Yellow fever, however, did not make its first appearance or attain its greatest severity in such places. Yellow fever was characteristically a coastal disease, located in or favoring ports engaged in frequent communication with infected tropical lands, and it maintained little or no sustained presence inland.[26] In contrast, paludism had been and could still be found wherever appropriate marsh conditions obtained, even in the middle of great continents.

Dutroulau pointed out that experience in the Antilles showed that yellow fever usually arrived in a dramatic, truly epidemic manner. The disease rapidly struck many persons in a previously healthy port or town and then disappeared, to return (if ever) after several seasons or to remain absent for years on end. The malarial fevers behaved differently: they seemed endemic to town or region, varying perhaps in intensity but rarely truly absent. In addition, lack of prior exposure — typical of new arrivals in a tropical port — was the strongest predisposition toward a severe case of yellow fever, whereas the longer an individual remained in a marshy region the greater became the risk of contracting paludal fever. Central to this conclusion was the observation, widely accepted by 1850 but denied earlier by Chervin and others, that "recidivism is the rule for paludal fevers but nonrecidivism holds for yellow fever."[27] Dutroulau held nonrecidivism, that is, the immune reaction provoked by yellow fever, to be a very important "differential character," one that clearly discriminated between the diseases in question.

Continuing his attack on Chervin's legacy, Dutroulau set out in parallel columns the primary symptoms of yellow fever and those of major forms of paludal or "pernicious" fever encountered in the tropics. "What could be more dissimilar," he asked, when contemplating his display, "than each of the three forms of pernicious fever that we have just described, when these are compared with yellow fever? What is more dissimilar than each of these forms when they are compared with one another, yellow fever

25. A. F. Dutroulau, "Fièvre jaune, sa spécificité, cas sporadiques," Archives générales de médecine, 5th ser., 1 (1853): 129–144, 433–449.

26. Dutroulau's comment reflects nineteenth-century experience and understanding of the disease; sylvan yellow fever and its nonhuman reservoirs were at the time unknown.

27. Dutroulau, "Fièvre jaune, sa spécificité, cas sporadiques," p. 137.

all the while remaining fundamentally the same, all of its characteristic signs being always observed, although these do vary in intensity?"[28] This faith in the unity and distinctness of yellow fever was confirmed by the final criterion for separating yellow fever and the paludal fevers: therapy. To Dutroulau, therapy, the "touchstone regarding the cause and nature of every disease," effected an indisputable separation. Quinine, as virtually everyone knew, acted as a specific remedy for the genuine paludal fevers; contrary, however, to what many believed or wanted to believe, it had no effect upon the victims of yellow fever, save when the latter suffered a concurrent case of malaria. In such a situation, the therapeutic effect was real, but the drug exercised no effect on the symptoms due to yellow fever.[29]

Dutroulau's characterization of yellow fever was built upon the dual basis of the clinical appearance and epidemiological behavior of the disease. Perhaps the specificity of yellow fever was not obvious to all observers and, certainly, when met in the isolated case, yellow fever could evoke great confusion. But by the 1850s, if not earlier, the medical profession in Europe as well as in the Americas was able to identify the disease even under highly unfavorable circumstances and could readily do so during pronounced epidemic outbreaks. Chervin's notion of a marsh- or filth-induced fever advancing by degrees towards its culmination in yellow fever was regarded as both false and dangerous: it was a constant invitation to misdiagnosis. In the case of yellow fever, confidence in identification was strengthened by the growing and well-founded skepticism of relying exclusively or even preponderantly upon supposedly pathognomonic signs such as black vomit or jaundice, neither present in all cases of the disease. Charles Belot, another student of the disease, stressed that in order to arrive at a yellow-fever diagnosis, the observer must seize both "the totality of the symptoms and the probabilities offered by local conditions."[30] Few could speak more authoritatively, for Belot had practiced medicine in Havana for several decades and fully appreciated the difficulties involved in diagnosing the disease.

The Saint-Nazaire epidemic was treated accordingly. Physicians examined suspected cases with great care and recognized that this disease was locally new. The overall disease situation was determined and observers found no grounds for concluding that the new disease was only the more acute condition of an endemic affliction. Hence, Saint-Nazaire, having been struck by a novel illness, had to seek the origin of its epidemic not within but without the town and region. After ruling out spontaneous generation and the bare (and ultimately irresponsible) claim that the event

28. Ibid., pp. 141–142.
29. Ibid., p. 143.
30. Charles Belot, *La fièvre jaune à la Havane. Sa nature et son traitement* (Paris: J. B. Baillière, 1865), p. 62.

was simply inexplicable, the remaining task was obvious to all: one must discover how the infection had entered the community. Confidence in the specificity of the disease and in the capacity to espy and describe that disease were crucial; without this foundation there would have been, literally, no object whose movement could be traced, and the entire investigation would have been in vain.[31]

What observers in Saint-Nazaire had seen and so carefully described was a very limited epidemic of yellow fever. The number of cases in the town and nearby ports was forty-one; of these victims, twenty-eight died.[32] These figures represent the epidemic *strictu sensu.* If to these numbers are added the sick (nine) and dead (two) aboard the *Anne-Marie* while in passage from Havana, the toll becomes fifty sick and thirty dead. The case-fatality rate ashore (68 percent), or even the 60 percent that includes the *Anne-Marie*, reveals the deadly effect of yellow fever moving through a susceptible population—although, as noted, these rates may be inflated due to neglect of subacute cases. During the course of the epidemic other ships also reached Saint-Nazaire from Havana, ships aboard which there was sickness, presumably yellow fever (four sick, of whom three died). It appears, however, that yellow fever did not move ashore from these later arrivals.

The epidemic reflected in figures presented, however, only the problem. There remained the important matter of how to counteract this intrusion of yellow fever. Sanitary action at Saint-Nazaire required, first of all, close scrutiny of the behavior of yellow fever within the community and renewed consideration of the origin and mode of transmission of the disease. The futility of therapy being recognized, it was evident that an exotic disease could be controlled only by refusing it access to a susceptible population. Mélier thus advanced from his principal conclusion—yellow fever is an imported disease—to the formulation and imposition of distinctive sanitary measures—a modified form of quarantine applicable to ships reaching France from yellow-fever ports. He also found himself caught up in reluctant and ultimately fruitless speculation on the cause of the disease.

31. A very few years later the same point was made with even greater force and now in regard to a dread disease that had repeatedly visited Europe, Asiatic cholera. Auguste Fauvel insisted categorically that the fact of disease specificity (and, presumably, also specific cause) was the only foundation upon which effective preventive action could be undertaken. See his *Le choléra. Etiologie et prophylaxie* (Paris: J. B. Baillière, 1868), pp. 18–22, a recapitulation, analysis, and development of the proceedings of the Constantinople International Sanitary Conference.

32. Counts of morbidity and mortality at Saint-Nazaire vary within Mélier's report. The following figures are based on the summary table in Mélier, "Relation de la fièvre jaune survenue à Saint-Nazaire," p. 124; each entry has been compared with the relevant "Pièce justificative." Mélier's own statement of mortality (ibid., p. 27) offers other figures.

4

Saint-Nazaire: Investigation and Action

*I*N SAINT-NAZAIRE few facts regarding public hygiene remained hidden from a determined inquirer. The town was small and events were well circumscribed. The investigator himself was thorough and the investigation timely. Mélier reported:

> It was easy for me in a place where everyone knows one another to learn with a certainty that the public health left nothing to be desired when the *Anne-Marie* arrived. The ship approached the town, she was received in the port, she was unloaded—and misfortune became evident. The relation between cause and effect, a relation which, rightly or wrongly, has been doubtful or obscure in other epidemics, is, in this epidemic, so patent and all the factual circumstances here are so well known, that one simply cannot comprehend how it could be possible to deny the importation [of the disease]. This [conclusion] is as clear as day and altogether incontestable.[1]

These confident and, it should be acknowledged, well-supported words answered one question, but they raised several others. The latter were the fundamental questions that concerned surveillance and sanitary control of the nation's frontiers.

Yellow Fever an Imported Disease

It had been Mélier's working hypothesis, just as it was to become his conclusion, that all cases of yellow fever at Saint-Nazaire took their "point of departure" from the *Anne-Marie*.[2] There were marked differences in the relationship between various victims and the ship, but exploration of these differences served only to confirm the essential connection. The first category of victims included men who had been in intimate contact with the *Anne-Marie*. Those most exposed were the stevedores who had unloaded the ship; the ship's second officer who had supervised discharge of the cargo;

---

1. François Mélier, "Relation de la fièvre jaune survenue à Saint-Nazaire en 1861," *Mémoires de l'Académie impériale de médecine* 26 (1863): 72.
2. Ibid., p. 28.

and Pierre Demais, a cooper who had spent many hours in the hold of the *Anne-Marie* repairing broken barrels. Mortality among the sick in this group approached 70 percent. Even worse was the experience of the unfortunate crew members of the *Chastang* who had visited the *Anne-Marie*, all five of whom subsequently died. Wishing to examine how the cargo of sugar had been stowed, they had not only breathed a contaminated atmosphere but handled the stalks of sugar cane used to secure the barrels and prevent shifting of the cargo. All of these men, Mélier noted, had been "plunged into the air within the ship and all received its direct action."[3]

The second category included less clear-cut cases. Here "immersion" in an infected atmosphere had not occurred, yet some form of influence had been transmitted. While naval discipline no doubt had prevented sailors from the *Cormoran* from boarding the *Anne-Marie*, the former ship nonetheless presented two victims of yellow fever. Men from the *Lorient No. 6* also probably did not board the *Anne-Marie*, although Mélier was less confident on this point. Nonetheless, that ship also exhibited yellow fever. In these instances, the disease influence appeared to act across a "more or less great distance," or by the victim "drawing near" to a source of infection.[4] Even if nothing else had been proved, the proximity of victim and infected ship was demonstrable.

It was the third category of victims that posed the more difficult but epidemiologically more interesting problems. Here facts were fewer and less sure, but one thing seemed certain: none of the victims had been aboard the *Anne-Marie* and apparently none had approached her. These persons contracted yellow fever by an "intermediary" means. Four such cases were cited, one of which was suspect and another was that of Alphonse Chaillon, his being the most remarkable case of the entire epidemic.

The first intermediate case was one of the two women struck by yellow fever. She was a seller of secondhand goods, identified only as "la femme Boquien." Mélier met this woman during or after her recovery, and he carefully examined her dwelling. He was assured that she had had no direct contact whatsoever with the *Anne-Marie* and had not approached the ship. Her trade and acquaintances, however, did establish a very tangible connection. In her shop she received two men from the crew of the *Anne-Marie* who brought with them used clothing, sail fragments, and old rope removed from their ship. Here was an "intermediary" or, rather, two intermediaries — men and fomites — that might explain Mme Boquien's sickness. The "very obscure" cause of the disease could have been borne by the men themselves or, as Mélier believed to be a more likely explanation,

3. Ibid., p. 29.
4. Ibid.

it might have been conveyed by the goods they brought with them, particularly the clothing. In any event, Mme Boquien's yellow fever, which appeared on 6 August, had been connected to the *Anne-Marie* even though the victim had not gone near the ship.[5]

Other evidence indicated that Mme Cadrier (*veuve* Ollivier) also had not been near the port. Her contact with men from the *Anne-Marie* was especially direct; she received them in her house or, as Mélier remarked, "probably in her bed." Her clients were the stevedores who were unloading the *Anne-Marie*. Sick on the seventh of August, Mme Cadrier was dead of yellow fever on the ninth. "Lacking any other explanation," the death of this fifty-five-year-old woman was assigned to contact with men who, compared to everyone else in the town, had been most exposed to the mysterious influence in the hold of the *Anne-Marie*.[6]

It appeared for a moment that the third case — that of the cobbler, René Bivault — would also suggest person-to-person contact or transmission by fomites. Bivault, who died of yellow fever on the tenth, was believed not to have been near the port or even to have left his shop. His only contact, therefore, would have been his assistant. In search of additional income, the latter helped unload the *Anne-Marie*. He worked in her hold and then returned in the evening in soaked clothing to the cobbler's shop. Closer inquiry revealed, however, that Bivault himself had visited the port. He had not boarded the *Anne-Marie*, but he had stood "downwind from her." This fact removed Bivault to the second category of influence and offered Mélier and others considerable relief.[7]

Bivault's case raises a question that might be posed regarding every victim of the epidemic. How did one know such things as wind direction, especially wind direction on earlier days and at specified hours? What else could be learned regarding the local meteorological situation? Remarkably enough, Saint-Nazaire was in this respect exceedingly well provided, possessing the most modern facilities for recording weather information. An engineer had been installed at Saint-Nazaire during the First Empire to observe and record the movement of tides; there was as yet no significant port. With the creation of the deep-water port and the rapid expansion of its activities under the Second Empire, this post was expanded. The office was charged with collecting comprehensive meteorological data, using the latest electrical recording equipment, and with maintaining a record of ship movements in the port. Using these records of wind direction, intensity, and duration, as well as reports of daily temperatures and

5. Ibid., pp. 29–30. The precise location of Mme Boquien's shop was not reported but it stood at a "certain distance" from the port.

6. Ibid., pp. 30–31.

7. Ibid., pp. 31–32.

of the position of shipping during the stay of the *Anne-Marie*, Mélier was able to prepare a topographico-meteorological history of the epidemic in the port area. Such facts, he knew, were not unfamiliar to the hygienic community. They had been used, when available, to decide the most suitable location of *lazarettos* and related sanitary installations. But, he proudly and properly announced, "rarely, so far as I know, have the facts been so clear as they are in this case and rarely have they been so well and so scientifically collected."[8] Data of such precision and comprehensiveness had never before been available for a European epidemic of yellow fever and perhaps for an epidemic of any disease. In this regard, Gibraltar in 1828 was a city without a history — a city that had collected no systematic meteorological information that could be incorporated into epidemiological analysis, and one that had preserved no useful record of the movement of shipping in her harbor.

Mélier's data revealed that all ships presenting yellow fever had, at least once during their stay in port, stood downwind, and close by, the *Anne-Marie*. Two ships, the *Chandarnagor* (see map location 3) and the *Lorient No. 8* (see map location 5), had docked near the *Anne-Marie*, but they escaped the fever. While in port, they had remained upwind from the infected vessel, from which Mélier concluded that no harmful influence could have been conveyed to their crew members.[9] Duration of wind movement was thought to be insignificant in comparison with wind direction and distance. But mere proximity did not assure transmission; an opposing wind had protected the *Chandarnagor*. And distance alone did not assure protection. The stonecutter, François Bruband, never approached the north side of the basin where the *Anne-Marie* was docked. Working near the entry channel (see map locations +B and B'), he remained at least seven hundred feet from the ship. On 4 August he fell ill; on the tenth he died, and yellow fever was the stated cause of death. It seemed evident that the wind had carried an infective principle across the harbor and delivered it with sufficient force to cause a fatal case of the disease.[10]

A good deal was known about the temperature limits of yellow fever. Obviously, the shock of meeting yellow fever in Saint-Nazaire, and soon afterward in Swansea, was all the greater because of the widely held belief that such relatively cool locations could not support the disease. Yellow fever had reached North Atlantic ports of Europe before, but rarely if ever had it come ashore and spread to persons unconnected with an infected ship. Between 26 July and 4 August, dates marking the arrival of the *Anne-*

8. Ibid., p. 34. Meteorological data from the onset of the epidemic (26 July–4 August) are reproduced in pièce 27, ibid., p. 224.

9. Ibid., p. 33.

10. Ibid., pp. 19, 34.

Marie and the onset of the epidemic, the average daily maximum temperature in Saint-Nazaire was 23.2°C; the highest single reading was 25.5°C on 1 August. The lows were cool indeed. The average low temperature for the same period was 14.4°C and the lowest single reading was 11.8°C on 28 July. Mélier drew no conclusions from these figures, but nineteenth-century observers knew that temperature did set limits to the entrance and spread of yellow fever, especially in the northern ports. The disease, it was believed, would not spread when temperatures fell below 20°C. However, if yellow fever had once gained a foothold, it was understood that only a frost could bring the outbreak to an end. No one had a satisfactory explanation for why this was so.[11]

Of the several instances of supposed "intermediate" transmission, it was the case of Alphonse Chaillon in Montoir that was most striking and, it appeared, most persuasive. If one could accept the available evidence, which seemed beyond dispute, only one conclusion was possible: yellow fever could be transmitted directly from a sick person to a susceptible one. Yellow fever was thus to be viewed as a contagious disease or, more precisely stated, yellow fever was *also* a contagious disease, for the case of Chaillon did nothing to diminish the well-supported notion of airborne transmission. What Mélier had in mind was not the transmutation of the disease during the course of an epidemic, as was proposed by contingent contagionist theory, but the possibility that one disease could move in two different ways. Such an interpretation would surely raise a number of new perplexities, but these Mélier did not address; the whole question of causation he found, and left, in sufficient confusion that this particular problem caused no undue difficulty.

Chaillon was a country physician who maintained a practice in the small village of Montoir, a station on the new railroad to Nantes and about four miles northeast of Saint-Nazaire.[12] Mélier reached Saint-Nazaire on 11 August and arranged immediately to hold regular conferences with local physicians, wishing thereby to have prompt word of all cases of illness in the region, including yellow fever. He learned from this group that Chaillon was treating at Montoir a number of the stevedores from the *Anne-Marie*

11. Ibid., p. 224. The extrinsic incubation period of yellow fever is markedly influenced by temperature, being greatly extended when the mosquito's ambient temperature falls below 25°C and perhaps impossible at sharply lower temperatures. Obviously, at Saint-Nazaire conditions were unfavorable for the perpetuation of the virus through more than one generation of the mosquitoes. See Loring Whitman, "The Arthropod Vectors of Yellow Fever," in *Yellow Fever*, ed. G. K. Strode (New York: McGraw-Hill, 1951), pp. 240–245; August Hirsch, *Handbook of Geographical and Historical Pathology*, 3 vols., trans. from the 2d German edition by Charles Creighton (London: New Sydenham Society, 1883–1886), 1:351–354.

12. Mélier, "Relation de la fièvre jaune survenue à Saint-Nazaire," pp. 35–41; pièce 13, pp. 160–164.

who had fallen ill. Chaillon was thus invited to attend the next conference in Saint-Nazaire. A note in reply from Mme Chaillon reported, however, that the doctor had suddenly fallen ill and could not travel. Mélier recalled his reaction to this news with distress. "I am surprised," he reported, "not to have been struck by this note. But at the time my tendency to accept the notion of nontransmission [that is, no person-to-person transmission], a notion which, nonetheless, I have never completely accepted, was such that, I confess no fear [for my colleague] was awakened."[13] Mélier never met Chaillon, for the latter, having taken seriously ill on the evening of 13 August, was dead of yellow fever late in the morning of the seventeenth.

No doubts arose regarding Chaillon's movements from the beginning of the epidemic until his death. He attended his patients in and near Montoir. He did not travel to Saint-Nazaire. He had "no connection, however remote, with the *Anne-Marie* or with any other vessel. It is equally certain that he neither saw nor touched any object of any kind that came from these ships or from the men who had been aboard them."[14] There remained, however, one connection with the port: the men themselves.

On 5 August, Chaillon was summoned to treat Alexis Briant for a disease whose seriousness the physician easily recognized. The following day he met the disease again, while caring for Théophile Ricordel, and soon thereafter while attending to Briant's father, Etienne. On the tenth, Chaillon began to treat Emile Poirier. All four men had worked in the hold of the *Anne-Marie*, all fell ill with yellow fever, and Ricordel and Poirier died of the disease, on the ninth and the fourteenth, respectively. Chaillon's contact with the ailing men was very close, the physician providing a massage when needed. Chaillon was of an excitable nature and, so it was said, prone to catch every disease that roamed the countryside. Even his outlook seemed negative. Upon hearing of the epidemic then spreading through Saint-Nazaire, he had announced that he, too, would probably catch that disease.

Whatever the powers of expectation, Chaillon did succumb to yellow fever, and to Mélier this sad event was a fact of "extreme importance" with regard to the question of transmission. On 16 August, the day before learning of Chaillon's fate, he had submitted a preliminary report and comments on his findings to the Ministry in Paris. He observed that the events at Saint-Nazaire

> confirm what I have said before, that is, up to the present time there have been no cases [of yellow fever] other than among persons who have been connected with the infected ship; none have been observed outside this bond.

13. Ibid., p. 37.
14. Ibid., p. 41.

Whether dead or convalescent, the afflicted individuals have communicated the disease to no one else. There have been no new cases either in the town or in the surrounding areas. . . . From all points of view, . . . from the scientific as well as the practical perspective, this fact is of the highest importance. It is easy for me to comprehend that if by some misfortune a contrary fact should present itself, we and particularly our consuls [abroad] will experience great uneasiness indeed.[15]

Chaillon constituted that very fact, and his case led Mélier to reflect earnestly and anew on the causation of yellow fever. He summarized the tendency of these reflections in the terse statement that it is now "very difficult not to see here a case of the transmission of yellow fever from person to person."[16]

On the one hand, the experience of Boquien, Cadrier, and especially Chaillon pointed to the contagious nature of yellow fever. On the other hand, analysis of the incidence of the disease in relation to wind direction and ship location reaffirmed the noncontagious character of yellow fever and suggested atmospheric transmission. The set of possibilities was not yet exhausted, however. Perhaps the infectious agent was conveyed by the ship's cargo. Mélier could deal summarily with this unwelcome suggestion. No evidence whatsoever appeared to indict the cargo aboard the *Anne-Marie*. Stevedores who had worked aboard the ship, breaking her carefully prepared stowage and moving the barreled sugar to dockside, had contracted yellow fever. Far more numerous, however, were the many workers who then conveyed those barrels to the nearby railroad, loaded them onto the cars, rode with them aboard the train to Nantes, saw to their removal from the train, and arranged them in the warehouse of the refiner. Careful inquiry revealed that none of these persons or any others with whom the workers or the barrels had come in contact manifested the least sign of yellow fever.[17] There was, therefore, no connection between yellow fever itself and the sugar and the wooden barrels in which it was contained, both of which had long resided in the doubtlessly infected hold of the *Anne-Marie*. Mélier thus absolved the ship's cargo, and by extension other such cargoes, from responsibility for the transmission of yellow fever. A quarter century earlier, the Academy of Medicine had reached the same conclusion during one of its more celebrated debates, then with reference to the spread of plague, especially by means of fomites.[18] These

15. Ibid., p. 36.
16. Ibid., p. 41.
17. Ibid., pp. 41–42.
18. R. C. Prus, *Rapport à l'Académie royale de médecine sur la peste et les quarantines, fait au nom d'une commission par M. le Dr. Prus*, 2 vols. (Paris: J. B. Baillière, 1846).

were sensitive matters, for it was important that needless suspicions not be raised when commercial activity was in question. Mere suspicion of the presence of infection could be almost as damaging as actual restraint of trade resulting from that suspicion. Cargo was the lifeblood of commerce; that blood was healthiest, and the nation's economic body strongest, when cargo moved regularly and rapidly, regardless of the condition of seamen, passengers, or ship.

An important fact at Saint-Nazaire thus turned out to be the "immunity," that is, the freedom from yellow fever, "of those persons who, *outside the ship*," had handled or otherwise approached the cargo discharged from the *Anne-Marie.*[19] Other observers had entertained the hypothesis of disease importation, exploring a variety of obvious modes of entry. Mélier also systematically considered and then eliminated one after another of these various possibilities. The example of Alphonse Chaillon certainly introduced a serious note of caution. If yellow fever were contagious, even to a very limited degree, then a familiar set of control measures, loosely called quarantine, seemed to be in order. Mélier, as will be seen, did take the possibility of contagion into consideration when devising his scheme of sanitary surveillance, but the latter was not based exclusively on this conclusion. He knew that ship's cargo posed no problem once it had been safely removed from the ship; the same was probably true of fomites, although their role, if any, did not become a significant issue at Saint-Nazaire.

Thus, if sick individuals played a very small and probably occasional role in the spread of the disease, and if a tainted cargo or other goods or objects played no role at all, there remained but one further possibility: the ship itself. She was infected, she bore the blame for the importation of the specific infection. Mélier made just this assignment, almost personifying the *Anne-Marie* and then ordering for her the application of extreme hygienic measures. The procedures employed were directed to the interior of the ship, to her structure, and to the enclosed air. The *Anne-Marie* was disinfected and the process, deemed a success at Saint-Nazaire, became the basis for a more general system of sanitary unloading, a system almost immediately introduced into French administrative rules and practice.

Sanitary Measures Proposed

There were two interrelated parts to Mélier's system of sanitary defense. Granting the possibility, if not probability, that a sick individual might be capable of importing yellow fever, it was necessary that all persons ar-

19. Mélier, "Relation de la fièvre jaune survenue à Saint-Nazaire," p. 42.

riving aboard a suspect vessel be subjected to a brief period of observation. Those who were not ill or did not become so could be safely released at the end of this period. The ship, containing an infectious miasma, itself required closer attention. She was given up to radical treatment. Banned from the harbor, she was subjected to thorough disinfection and cleansing. Only after careful inspection could she be returned to her owner and reenter service. This process Mélier called sanitary unloading, and he made it the centerpiece of his proposed protective measures.

His objective was to reassert sanitary control over the nation's frontiers and to do so in a scientific manner. Control did *not* mean a return to the harsh and inflexible measures popularly regarded as the essence of traditional quarantine. Mélier's science, epidemiology, taught that one could seek protection without recourse to arbitrary practices.

Quarantine in the mid-nineteenth century possessed an evil reputation. To proud, modern ears it rang of medieval barbarism, worthy perhaps of Levantine nations (whose hygienic arrangements Europeans rarely admired) but hardly suited to the civilized tastes of so-called progressive Westerners. When vigorously enforced, quarantine disrupted the entire life of a community or nation. Of course, the most serious damage, or so critics claimed, was done to commerce and thus to the economic foundations of town and state. And there was a further and really unanswerable complaint: quarantine and its close relative, the sanitary cordon, in most cases simply did not work. Their ineffectiveness had been demonstrated on repeated occasions, the plague coming ashore or across the continent from the east no matter what measures were taken to prevent its arrival. Asiatic cholera, too, passed all barriers.

Quarantine had been introduced in the fourteenth and fifteenth centuries. It was based on earlier practices aimed at isolating the leper, but was then directed against the plague, whose first massive outbreak in 1347–1348 marked a turning point in the affairs of medieval society. Gradually, the use of quarantine spread across Europe from the ports and cities of the western Mediterranean littoral. Quarantine laws and practices have differed greatly in different countries and have also changed with time. No less important, these measures have been enforced with varying degrees of severity and often, despite being the law of the land, not enforced at all.

There is no general history of quarantine, and for good reason.[20] The

20. Léon Colin, "Quarantines," *Dictionnaire encyclopédique des sciences médicales,* 100 vols. (Paris: Victor Masson, P. Asselin, 1869–1889), 80:3–171. Also François Hildesheimer, "La protection sanitaire des côtes françaises au XVIIIᵉ siècle," *Revue d'histoire moderne et contemporaine* 27 (1980): 443–467; Gavin Milroy, "Historical Sketch of Quarantine Legislation and Practice in Great Britain," *Parliamentary Papers* 58 (1861) [Accounts and Papers.

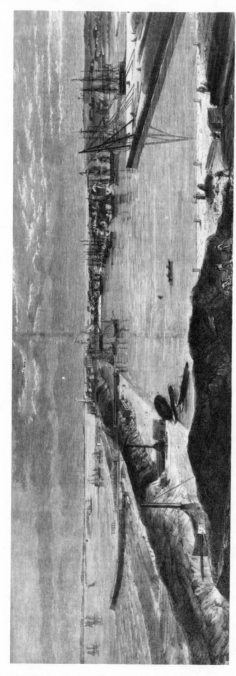

Construction of the first tidal port at Saint-Nazaire, middle 1850s. To the left, the new dike against the sea and the connecting canal; in the left background stands the old fishing town, with ships tied to the Old Mole. To the right, behind the shipping already using the unfinished port, rises the new town. The *Anne-Marie* in 1861 stood just behind the crane on the right. (Courtesy of the Ecomusée de Saint-Nazaire.)

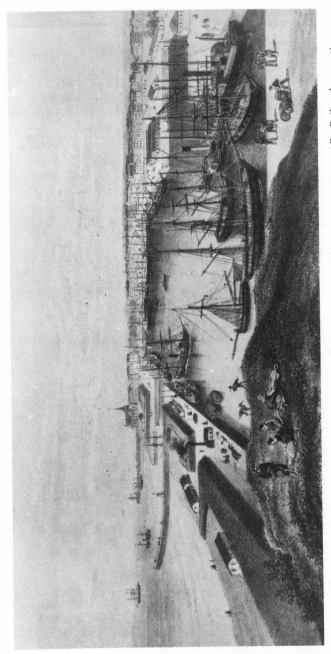

The completed port, again viewed from the north, with quais fully developed and the new town growing rapidly. Railroad connections were established just beyond the quai on the near right. (Courtesy of the Ecomusée de Saint-Nazaire.)

subject exhibits numerous and large national variations and a singular in-
ventiveness that showed itself best with the appearance of any new threat.
It also presents in uncommonly striking manner the eternal contradiction
between the stated terms of the law and how nations and individuals actually conduct their affairs under the law. A quarantine law on the books
was often just that and nothing more. Sometimes the law was only permissive; a response to the threat of disease might or might not be made.
Such was the British quarantine law of 1825. The law — or commonly the
administrative regulation or royal edict — might, however, require that action be taken. And sometimes it was. Often enough, when action was taken,
not all measures envisaged were put into effect or enforced with equal vigor.
Quarantine and cordons were expensive and merchants and port authorities frequently failed to provide the funds needed to assure effective procedures. Quarantine and, especially, cordons required large-scale and often
complex organizational activity, usually involving military force and
reaching into the most remote corners of the nation. Leakage through the
barriers was common and could be significant. One must, therefore, approach the subject with great caution, for the written history of quarantine is generally a history of legislation and of proposed or promised efforts.
It rarely deals with how a given quarantine was put into effect, the fate
of the community thus isolated, and the beneficial or fatal consequences
of the measures taken.[21]

Critics and popular thought both tended to see quarantine as an inflexible monolith, which no doubt it could be. The word, however, acquired and has preserved a generic meaning, embracing a range of measures
used to control the movement of men, goods, and ships in international
ports. In its most rigid form, all three arrivals would be isolated and
prevented from making any contact with the new port and its hinterland.
The period of isolation might be the traditional forty days, but it could
also be considerably shorter. If disease was present among arriving crewmen or passengers, or, perhaps even more important, if disease was still
only latent in this population, it would have an opportunity under quarantine to declare itself and run its course during isolation. The healthy, or
survivors, might then be free to come ashore. During this period, too, the
potentially harmful influence thought to be carried by cargo or fomites

25. Shipping and Trade. No. 544. Papers Relating to Quarantine communicated to the Board
of Trade on the 30th Day of July 1861]: 39–48; William Collinridge, "On Quarantine," *Lancet*
2 (1897): 715–721, 787–792, 863–868; C. F. Mullett, "A Century of English Quarantine," *Bulletin of the History of Medicine* 23 (1949): 527–545; and esp. J. C. McDonald, "The History
of Quarantine in Britain during the 19th Century," ibid., 25 (1951): 22–44.

    21. But see Carlo Cipolla, *Christofano and the Plague. A Study of the History of Public
Health in the Age of Galileo* (Berkeley: University of California Press, 1973).

could be reduced or dissipated by exposure of these goods to the atmosphere either on deck or in isolated and carefully guarded warehouses. Full quarantine was rightly thought to be an arduous, annoying, expensive, and dangerous affair.

The history of quarantine during the nineteenth century is marked by a continuing effort to minimize the rigors of isolation and by a recognition that quarantine should no longer be thought of simply as a regularized set of practices to be directed against the threat of exotic disease. The latter contributed greatly to the former. By 1820 yellow fever had been added to plague as a disease thought to require quarantine; Asiatic cholera joined this short list after 1830. These were the classic nineteenth-century pestilential diseases, those over which the battle regarding importation and local causes raged, and those which provided rich opportunities for the contagionist-noncontagionist disputes. But plague, because of its long absence, was only occasionally brought into these discussions; among the exotic diseases, cholera and yellow fever stood at the center of epidemiological and etiological dispute. Quarantine (and it proved difficult to avoid both the word and the centuries-old usages associated with it) was forced to fit these diseases, that is, it became increasingly disease-specific. Protective measures were to be adjusted, so far as knowledge allowed, to the distinctive epidemiological character of the disease in question. The inquiry conducted at Saint-Nazaire and the preventive measures devised and implemented there by Mélier made an important contribution to these developments.

France, like the other European nations, had no easy time seeking a coherent national quarantine policy. It was not until the 1850s that sanitary surveillance of ports and frontiers was relegated to a clearly defined central administrative authority. In 1822, the government had approved legislation that extended to all of France the severe measures against imported disease that local authorities in Marseilles had kept ever at the ready. Should a threat arise, the new law authorized widespread intervention in the movement of persons and goods. It was this law of 3 March 1822 — together with what was perceived to be the mentality that had assured its passage and the primitive machinery that would presumably be used to enforce it — that had so provoked Chervin and the noncontagionist party and that led to two decades of bitter medicopolitical controversy.[22]

These interminable disputes undermined attempts to put the quarantine provisions of the law into effect. Outside of Marseilles, where fear

---

22. The text of this law is reproduced in Colin, "Quarantines," pp. 44–46. Events after 1822 have been closely examined: see E. H. Ackerknecht, "Anticontagionism between 1821 and 1867," *Bulletin of the History of Medicine* 22 (1948): 562–593. The passage and political

of plague was still alive despite no recent approaches, the desire to try to impose quarantines and sanitary cordons in threatening situations had declined greatly by the mid-1830s and remained in extreme disfavor through the 1840s.[23] But the law of 1822 remained in force.

When Asiatic cholera moved across Europe in 1830–1832, local and national authorities in many countries attempted to halt its progress by the imposition of quarantine in the ports and of sanitary cordons ashore. Neither measure stopped or even slowed the advance of the disease. Informed opinion concluded and long supported the notion that such measures were either impotent or unenforceable and probably both. When the threat of cholera returned in the later 1840s, so did these reservations. However, the protective potential of full or partial quarantine was thought to deserve at least some reconsideration.

An important step in clarifying the situation was the convening at the request of the French government of the first International Sanitary Conference.[24] The conference members — twelve European nations sent delegations each consisting of one diplomat and one physician — met in Paris in the summer of 1851. Mélier, acting in his newly acquired role of Inspector General of Sanitary Services, established the topics for discussion. Cholera was the principal concern of this and the many succeeding sanitary conferences. Plague was not forgotten and yellow fever, too, received some consideration. Neither, however, posed the present and alarming peril that cholera did.

Discussion centered on the question of the efficacy or inefficacy of quarantine measures against Asiastic cholera and whether such measures should be (re)introduced. Needless to say, opinion was sharply divided and the issue was resolved, in the usual manner and on paper at least, by a vote. Of the twenty-three delegates voting, fifteen agreed that cholera should be subject to quarantine, four opposed this view, and four abstained. In the opposition stood two very worried interests: Britain, who sought to maximize freedom of trade; and Turkey, whose dominance of the Levan-

---

manipulation of this law are vividly portrayed by G. D. Sussman, "From Yellow Fever to Cholera. A Study of French Government Policy, Medical Professionalism, and Popular Movements in the Epidemic Crises of the Restoration and the July Monarchy" (New Haven: Ph.D. diss., Yale University, 1971), pp. 131–183.

23. Still in 1850, Mélier thought it wise to soften up a Marseilles audience with promises of new and reasonable laws, at the same time offering laudatory words on the dedication of a new *lazaretto* in that city: *Ouverture du Lazaret de Ratoneau. Discours prononcé par M. le docteur Mélier* (Marseilles: Barlatier-Feissat-Demonchy, 1850). The city's concern was well founded; she had suffered an extraordinary epidemic of plague a century earlier; see C. Carrière et al., *Marseille ville morte. La peste de 1720* (Marseilles: M. Gargon, 1968).

24. Norman Howard-Jones, *The Scientific Background of the International Sanitary Conferences, 1851–1938* (Geneva: World Health Organization, 1975), pp. 9–16.

tine ports was a critical matter to all trading nations, including herself. The deliberations of the conference were binding on no nation and no real action followed upon the meeting, except in France.

The French took seriously the notion that Asiatic cholera was a pestilential disease. It was at this time that it officially joined plague and yellow fever in this select category. The conference spurred Mélier and his associates to redesign and expand the provisions of the quarantine law of 1822. This they quickly did, and their efforts were rewarded by the promulgation of an Imperial decree, a fundamental document in the history of quarantine in France. The sanitary decree of 1853 confirmed that nation's adherence to an "international sanitary convention concluded between France, Sardinia and various other maritime powers."[25] In truth, no other powers ratified the convention. It did not become an instrument for coordinated international activity in matters of quarantine, but it did offer a reasoned program that could be used as a guide for further investigation or as a model for legislative or administrative innovation.

The convention and decree of 1853 were seen to offer France a great advantage in sanitary matters. At very least, she now possessed a comprehensive body of law and administrative regulations pertaining to the quarantine question. The British quarantine act of 1825 had created no standardized practice and provided no assurance of regular and competent administrative authority. It was, as noted, only a permissive act. Opposition to quarantine was as strong in Britain as it was in France. Moreover, the act assigned quarantine responsibilities to local authorities, who might or might not apply the needed measures, which they themselves were to devise.[26] To be effective, quarantine required much broader competencies than these. In France, too, local sanitary action proved extremely difficult to implement, and local interests commonly prevailed over cen-

25. Ibid., pp. 15–16. The text of the convention of 27 May 1853 is reproduced in Colin, "Quarantines," pp. 60–71, and in Ambroise Tardieu, "Sanitaire (Régime)," *Dictionnaire d'hygiène publique et de salubrité*, 2d ed., 4 vols. (Paris: J. B. Baillière, 1862), 3:54–76. To the convention and the decree issued a few days later were added a series of detailed "Instructions sur l'exécution du décret du 4 juin 1853 sur la police sanitaire": these instructions are not reproduced by Colin but appear in Tardieu, "Sanitaire (Régime)," pp. 76–97. It should be noted that the "decree" of 1853 actually consists of two independent but interrelated parts, the first being the "sanitary convention" concluded between France and the Kingdom of Sardinia on 27 May 1853 and the second being the above "instructions" together with Napoleon's orders that gave the convention the force of law in France and indicated how the stated provisions were to be applied, this second part bearing the date of 4 June 1853.

26. See McDonald, "History of Quarantine in Britain," pp. 36–38, who also notes the singular fact that Parliament in 1866, when approving the Sanitary Act of that year, provided a second and independent piece of hygienic legislation that contradicted important provisions of the 1825 Act; the latter continued in force.

tral initiative. But defense of the frontier was an avowedly national concern and here the central government more easily assumed a commanding role.

The French decree of 1853 was silent on scientific matters, taking no formal stand on the disruptive themes of contagion and noncontagion. The decree was also a conservative document, largely reflecting the expectation and practice of quarantine in the Mediterranean ports; it contained no novelties regarding disease theory or even hygienic routine. But, as Léon Colin insisted in 1889, France had in fact acquired a comprehensive sanitary law and, most important, it was a law that contained little to antagonize contending medical opinions or other rival interests. This was a novel and very promising contribution, and it became the foundation for the development of sanitary controls in the French ports. It was a foundation that could be expanded or amended as new knowledge became available or new needs arose. In the French case, law provided flexibility and allowed an escape from the ad hoc responses, or the failure to respond, that too often characterized the efforts of local authorities facing an impending epidemic.

The decree also gave form to the hastily renewed organization of national sanitary authority. Here again events immediately preceding the conference had played a major role. In 1848 quarantine against cholera had been abolished, against fierce opposition in the Mediterranean ports. The measure was reestablished in 1850, whereby France created a series of local health councils in all of her maritime departments. Administrative and military officers, local dignitaries, customs officials, and physicians served on these councils. Three years later, Article 102 of the sanitary decree created the post of Director of Sanitary Services, a position which, under other designations and with varied attributions, Mélier had obtained in 1850 and which he would retain until his death. Article 103 defined the functions of this position. The senior responsible officer of the national sanitary service, the director was "to oversee the execution of sanitary laws and regulations, determine or have determined the sanitary condition of arriving ships, deliver bills of health to departing ships, and exercise direction and surveillance over lazarettos and quarantine ports."[27] In these roles he could draw upon the advice of the reconstituted local health councils (articles 104–109). The latter played only an advisory role; final authority in all matters rested with the director of sanitary services or his delegate. The new sanitary establishment—both a rationalization of and an unprecedented improvement upon French maritime sanitary practice—was also a visible expression of the far-reaching authority of the new empire.

27. Colin, "Quarantines," pp. 68–69.

Mélier in Paris and soon thereafter in Saint-Nazaire exploited fully the new regulations. As director of sanitary services, he was by law a member of the Saint-Nazaire health council, and when in the port city he met regularly with its members, obtaining information regarding the epidemic and the sanitary condition of the region. After taking this varied information and advice into consideration, he determined what measures were to be imposed and ensured that they were in fact implemented. In determining these measures, he began by following the guidelines that had emerged at the Sanitary Conference of 1851 and then formed part of the decree of 1853.

A supposition of the law of 1822 was that quarantine was an efficacious means of halting or at least reducing the damage done by a pestilential disease. That supposition persisted, although it could not and did not determine sanitary action in an era in which the force of the law was regularly diminished by royal decrees and changing administrative rules. By the 1850s, however, understanding of the measures necessary for effective quarantine or, better, for hygienic protection of the nation, was beginning rapidly to deepen.

Colin rightly emphasized the great importance of this change, especially the significance of the growing recognition that quarantine must be made disease-specific. Quarantine measures, he observed,

> those now in effect and especially those stated in the regulation of 1853, most certainly will not be applied with the same chances of success to the different pestilential diseases. Among these diseases there are some wherein the danger of transmission is much greater and longer lasting and which render ineffective or less useful the protective measures that work well against other diseases. It follows that it would be unreasonable to condemn broadly or to exalt beyond measure quarantine practices only on the basis of their favorable or unfavorable effect upon a single such disease. . . . The rules established by tradition no doubt would provide, thanks to their uniformity, great ease in their application; but to impose these unchanging rules when climate and local conditions are very different and when the nature of the epidemic disease which we seek to halt is also quite different, is to act in defiance of the knowledge that science has today given us.[28]

Colin's vast essay on quarantine is a celebration of the contribution of science to the study of pestilential disease and its prevention. He rebuked those who argued only on the basis of inherited practice or confined themselves to arguing once again the rival merits of contagionism and noncontagionism. The science in question was a new one, epidemiology, and its

28. Ibid., pp. 90, 6.

practitioners, whom he comfortably called epidemiologists, were those physicians who had made "a special study of diseases of exotic origin" and thus were responsible for the decisive new understanding of the distinctiveness of these diseases.[29]

Colin had argued partially within the framework of a private polemic, but his point is a broader and an important one. He was a sharp critic of Louis Pasteur and the more enthusiastic advocates of the germ theory of disease and also a well-informed epidemiologist (his *Traité des maladies épidémiques* was published in 1879). Just like case-tracing, disease specificity was not a new idea. Even in connection with the particular problem of quarantine, both notions had been expressed and also employed since at least the sixteenth century. But the idea of disease specificity had been greatly extended and rendered more precise during the early nineteenth century, this being the fundamental contribution of the clinician and pathologist to the new science of epidemiology. Disease specificity was especially important in the large and confusing realm of "fevers," a category now shown to be an assemblage of many distinct disease entities. Among fevers were some that had rarely caused confusion; their distinctive traits were either obvious or easily established and the specific disease also readily identified. Such was the case of smallpox and epidemic forms of plague. But there were other fevers that only later acquired a well-drawn and stable clinical identity. Among these are many of mankind's most common and feared afflictions and some that are less common but no less fatal. Yellow fever belonged to this latter category, as did Asiatic cholera.

Given these regulations and this new scientific understanding, what was to be done in Saint-Nazaire? As noted earlier, examination of the role of the *Anne-Marie* in the epidemic at Saint-Nazaire indicated clearly that persons *outside the ship* (with the exception of Chaillon and a few others) did not contract yellow fever. A connection between men and ship had been suspected by others, and Mélier was not the first to cast suspicion on the *Anne-Marie*. On orders from an apprehensive local health council, she had been removed from the quai on 5 August and anchored in the middle of the northern arm of the basin (see map location A), some two hundred feet from the nearest ship. Two days later she was taken from the basin and placed in the roadstead of Saint-Nazaire. Even this seemed insufficient. Mélier's first action after meeting with the health council was to order the *Anne-Marie* towed to the roadstead at Mindin, across the Loire, there to be secured in total isolation.[30]

The health council and the government's sanitary inspector obviously

29. Ibid., p. 107.
30. Mélier, "Relation de la fièvre jaune survenue à Saint-Nazaire," p. 44.

agreed on a basic working hypothesis — the likelihood of an infected ship — and they did so before an exhaustive analysis of the epidemic was completed. This hypothesis, which such analysis then confirmed, guided all subsequent prophylactic undertakings. While the *Anne-Marie* awaited further attention, Mélier addressed the closely related problem of the potential epidemic influence of her scattered crew members. These men, who were inscribed with the maritime administration, were traced to their homes; none was reported ill. This fact, which was only to be expected, made the fate of the stevedores, new men who had boarded the *Anne-Marie*, all the more striking.

Granting, then, the infected condition of the *Anne-Marie*, a sanitary attack on the ship was clearly in order. Needed were selective but thorough disinfection and short-term but absolute isolation. Cargo such as the barreled sugar that the *Anne-Marie* carried had been shown to pose no threat when once removed from the ship. Indeed, the very act of removal itself worked a sanitary effect. "Once merchandise has been removed from the hold and, as the saying goes, one has *broken cargo*, whatever disease germs or principles are in question are promptly dissipated and perhaps even destroyed; from this it follows that it would be superfluous to observe much used, and abused, precautions, that is, rigorous quarantine."[31] Of course, the act of unloading a ship posed a hazard to those who worked aboard her. The fate of the stevedores at Saint-Nazaire proved the truth of this long-standing proposition once and for all. It seemed indispensable, during the unloading process, to disinfect each stowed object before it was moved and to maintain throughout the ship strong defenses against the infective influence.

Disinfection was thus to be directed at the irreducible *foyer d'infection*, the ship itself. Yet the ship was really only the vehicle of the infection, which in turn was surely a noxious influence that moved with the air or was perhaps a corrupted species of air. As such, it was carried within the ship and could penetrate, as could ordinary atmospheric air, deeply into the very structure of the ship.

One of the striking conclusions drawn from the Saint-Nazaire epidemic was the definition of just which air was involved in the transmission of yellow fever. It was not, as Chervin and others maintained, a peculiar local condition of the atmosphere, one due to a peculiar corrupting influence that had arisen from changed and deleterious local conditions. Not at all: this poisonous air had come aboard a ship in Havana. (How had it come to be present in Havana? Mélier did not pose this question and thus avoided a potentially infinite regression of questions.) It had then crossed the sea

31. Ibid., pp. 59–60.

in a small sailing ship, apparently scarcely able to pass beyond deck and planking, and it was the cause of yellow fever. It was indeed a common cause, standing at the origin of a specific disease that was the same on both sides of the ocean. Specificity of cause went hand in hand with specificity of disease.

Common to both Mélier and Chervin was the conviction that, since infected air was the principal (according to Mélier) or exclusive (according to Chervin) agent responsible for yellow fever, the best countermeasure was atmospheric disinfection. Chervin's view dictated communitywide sanitation, a campaign directed at obvious hygienic nuisances. It also entailed, when authorities recognized that their campaign was not halting the epidemic, the forced movement of large populations to what were hoped to be more healthful areas. In 1828 the population of whole districts of Gibraltar was moved to presumably safe ground. By stating that the source of yellow fever had been imported aboard the *Anne-Marie*, Mélier's general conclusion redefined and thereby limited the field of sanitary intervention.

The purpose of disinfection is, of course, to counteract the influence of an infection. The latter has acquired many meanings over the centuries, but nineteenth-century usage (tied closely to the doctrine of noncontagion) continued to stress the idea of an atmospherically borne poison.[32] The atmosphere receives from various sources noxious substances, which it then conveys to susceptible human beings. A foul or unusual odor is the first sign of the presence of such an infection. Disinfection obviously reverses this chain of thought and action. "A body is called a disinfectant," wrote Pierre Chalvet in a comprehensive review of the question (1863), "when it possesses the property of removing from the air or from any material whatsoever, noxious qualities that have been acquired through impregnation by extremely subtle substances of diverse natures (these are called miasmata, emanations or effluvia)." Chalvet, a Parisian physician, had explored a wide range of chemical disinfectants and had a definite prophylactic program in mind.

> We also call disinfectants those bodies that can destroy the fetid elements that arise under the influence of the putrid decomposition of once-living organized bodies. . . . Chemical disinfectants are those that form imputrescible combinations with the organic matter of wounds or the products of putrefaction. Under ordinary conditions these combinations can form neither new miasmata nor recreate exhalations that have already been destroyed.[33]

32. See Owsei Temkin, "An Historical Analysis of the Concept of Infection," in *The Double Face of Janus and Other Essays in the History of Medicine* (Baltimore: Johns Hopkins University Press, 1977), pp. 456–471.

33. Pierre Chalvet, "Des désinfectants et de leurs applications à la thérapeutique et à l'hygiène," *Mémoires de l'Académie impériale de médecine* 26 (1863): 473–476.

Chalvet's view followed closely the chemical view of disease causation characteristic of the period. This theory assigned the predominant role in the origin of disease and support of morbid processes to distinct chemical, nonliving substances. These substances, having made contact with organic matter under appropriate conditions, launched a series of disaggregative molecular motions that led to the disruption of organic functions and ultimately to the dissolution of the bodily frame.[34] An effective disinfectant might thus be a substance that possessed the virtue of joining with organic molecules and forming combinations that were no longer subject to putrefaction or other degradation; it might also purge the atmosphere of the threatening substance.

The disinfection of the *Anne-Marie* and of later ships arriving from Havana was to be led by chlorine. This element, variously combined or in the gaseous state, was used widely in the early nineteenth century for the treatment of wounds and for various prophylactic undertakings. Discovered in 1774, chlorine provided the active agent for the muriatic fumigations that the medical world viewed as a potent means to control the spread of infection. Such measures were also applied during the early European yellow-fever and other epidemics but were thought to have given only equivocal or unsatisfactory results.

Chalvet in 1863 hoped to persuade the medical community of the importance of regular use of chemical disinfectants, especially in hospital practice. Among these substances, chlorinated compounds were again preferred. Chalvet stressed the well-established and more far-reaching use of chlorine as a general prophylactic measure. Its use in hospitals was emphasized, and for good reason: the 1850s and 1860s witnessed the rapid and deadly spread of hospital-induced disease, in response to which numerous investigations were conducted and new procedures introduced, especially surgical procedures conducted under antiseptic and aseptic conditions.[35] Chalvet's hygienic program for the hospital was simplicity itself.

34. This was the interpretation of the process of "infection" introduced by Justus von Liebig in the late 1830s and continued by him and others into the new era of the germ theory of disease. See Liebig, *Chemische Briefe*, Wohlfeile Ausgabe (Leipzig and Heidelberg: C. F. Winter, 1865), pp. 178–189; Margaret Pelling, *Cholera, Fever and English Medicine, 1825–1865* (Oxford: Oxford University Press, 1978), pp. 113–145. Also Wilhelm Griesinger, *Infectionskrankheiten, Malariakrankheiten, gelbes Fieber, Typhus, Pest, Cholera* [Rudolf Virchow, ed., *Handbuch der speciellen Pathologie und Therapie*, Bd. II, 2te Abtheilung], 2d ed. (Erlangen: F. Enke, 1864), p. 3; John Farley, *The Spontaneous Generation Controversy. From Descartes to Oparin* (Baltimore: Johns Hopkins University Press, 1977), pp. 47–50, 85.

35. It was recognized that disinfection works best if directed against the "insalubrious and dangerous matter itself"—but the existence of this matter was only suspected and its nature was utterly unknown: Antoine Fauvel, *Le choléra. Etiologie et prophylaxie* (Paris: J. B. Baillière, 1868), pp. 384–414. On noscomial disease or hospitalism, see Hirsch, *Geographical*

A hospital hall should smell of chlorine or have no smell at all! We believe that, because of the large number of persons gathered there, it may be advantageous [constantly] to maintain chlorine vapor in its atmosphere. And if hygienic principles are rigorously followed, one will see that the walls and ceilings of these halls are whitewashed each year and after every epidemic. It is also advisable to have spare halls that can be successively occupied and thus favor an annual *expurgation* [using chlorine].[36]

Chalvet dealt with the hospital, Mélier with a ship. Both objects, however, presented tightly closed spaces rampant with airborne infection, and it is not surprising that the two physicians adopted the same prophylactic measures. There was nothing novel in Mélier's disinfection procedures, save the thoroughness with which they were applied to an infected ship.

Sanitary Measures Imposed

The *Anne-Marie* now lay anchored off the left bank of the Loire several miles from Saint-Nazaire. She had already killed many men and was thought to be capable of taking the lives of still others. Earlier practice in dealing with such vessels was often extreme: local port authorities would seize the ship and immediately sink her, or, the ultimate solution, she would be burned with her cargo still aboard. A significant objective of the Sanitary Conference of 1851 was to find means to avoid these harsh and expensive, if perhaps effective, hygienic measures. In such matters, Mélier emphasized, experts must seek to "reconcile the two interests that are involved . . . that of [public] health first of all and then that of the property owner. The latter interest, while no doubt much less significant than the former, nonetheless possesses a real importance because often it constitutes the very well-being of the shipowner and his associates."[37]

The *Anne-Marie*, being a sound if unhealthy ship, was therefore to be saved. The rescue constituted Mélier's modification of quarantine regulations for yellow fever.[38] The ship was beached in shallow water at high

and Historical Pathology 2:389–491; Jules Chauvel, "Pourriture d'hôpital," *Dictionnaire encyclopédique des sciences médicales* 79:350–361; Edmond Boisseau, "Hôpitaux," ibid., 50: esp. pp. 290–304 ("Influences noscomiales"); K. C. Carter, "Translator's Introduction," in Ignaz Semmelweis, *The Etiology, Concept and Prophylaxis of Childbed Fever*, trans. and ed. K. C. Carter (Madison: University of Wisconsin Press, 1983), pp. 3–58; W. W. Cheyne, *Lister and His Achievement* (London: Longmans, Green, 1925), pp. 39–71; O. H. Wangensteen et al., "Surgical Cleanliness, Hospital Salubrity and Surgical Statistics, Historically Considered," *Surgery* 71 (1972): 477–493.

36. Chalvet, "Désinfectants et leurs applications," p. 551.
37. Mélier, "Relation de la fièvre jaune survenue à Saint-Nazaire," p. 45.
38. Ibid., pp. 46–49; pièce 14D, pp. 166–171. The various elements of Mélier's scheme

tide. Fifty kilograms of iron sulfate, a substance thought to be particularly effective in neutralizing corrupted organic matter, were cast into the hold. The next day a series of openings was made in the lower hull. The *Anne-Marie* remained in this situation for eight full days, the iron sulfate being swept over her inner planking and her foul hold being repeatedly flushed by the large tides at the mouth of the river. Having already been unloaded, her valuable cargo was not endangered. There was, however, one difficulty: no local laborers would go near the ship to perform the necessary operations. A detachment from the Imperial Navy overcame this problem. Since direct treatment of the innards of the ship was the central element in this process of hygienic scuttling (*sabordement*), careful disinfection had to precede and accompany every movement. Human contact with the interior of the ship, including the debris, sand, and miscellaneous filth that she contained, was not allowed without a chlorine preparation being first applied to the material in question. Even the massive ballast stones were disinfected. Once the rubbish was removed, the ship was flushed with clean water.

The *Anne-Marie* was scuttled on 13 August. The holes in her hull then being closed, she was raised on the twenty-fifth and meticulous cleaning of the ship's structure begun. This was completed on 11 September. A week was required for drying. Finally, after five weeks of attention, the ship was ready to be returned to her owner on 19 September. The *Anne-Marie* had been the cause of a remarkable epidemic and she deservedly commanded exceptional sanitary attention. This system might be effective but, being slow and expensive, it placed a great burden on port facilities, which were usually inadequate to the task. *Sabordement* and timber-by-timber cleansing seemed hardly suited to routine protection from imported pestilential disease.

And in 1861 such disease continued to arrive. Fourteen ships reached Saint-Nazaire from Cuba between 3 August (when the *Etoile de la mer* from Havana followed the *Anne-Marie* into port) and 15 September. Most were sailing vessels carrying sugar, most were as filthy and damp within

---

of sanitary unloading had been proposed and sometimes used by others; see, for example, Paul Carsar, *Medical History of Malta* (London: Wellcome Historical Medical Library, 1964), pp. 285–297. Around 1860, these elements were being brought together to form a set of "new" approaches to quarantine by persons other than Mélier; the conclusions reached were often similar. William Bryson and especially Gavin Milroy proposed an "English system" of quarantine (McDonald, "History of Quarantine in Britain", pp. 35–36); the parallels with Mélier's scheme were close but the incubation period was not emphasized and cleansing of the ship was largely ignored. More vigorous intervention was apparently contemplated by Joseph Holt in the United States: Margaret Warner, "Hunting the Yellow Fever Germ: The Principle and Practice of Etiological Proof in Late Nineteenth-Century America," *Bulletin of the History of Medicine* 59 (1985): 361–382.

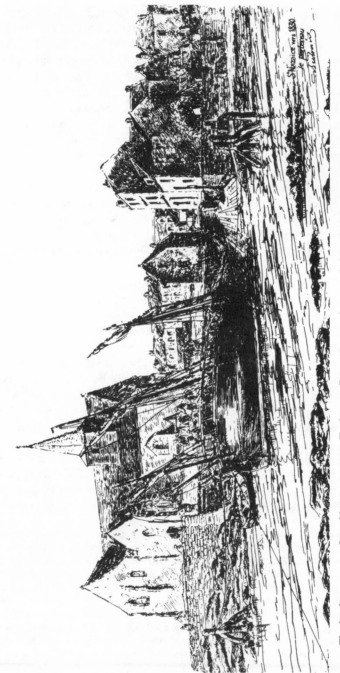

The landing stage at Saint-Nazaire in 1830. To this small "port" came the coastal shipping, always of slight tonnage, that constituted the town's contact with the maritime world prior to the opening of the great new port in 1856. (Gaston Le Floc'h and Fernand Guériff, *Saint-Nazaire* [*Loire-Atlantique, 44*] [Colmar-Ingersheim: Editions S.A.E.P., 1974], p. 44.)

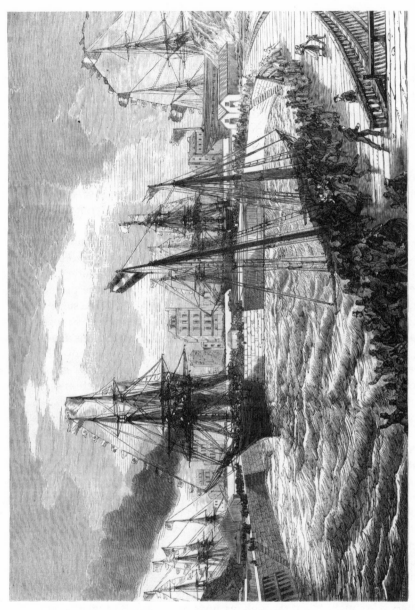

Saint-Nazaire in her early glory. The *Louisiane* sails for Mexico on 14 April 1862, inaugurating regular transatlantic service between France and that country and the entire Caribbean area. The yellow-fever ship, the *Anne-Marie*, had stood, two years earlier, directly across the port behind the *Louisiane*. (*Le monde illustré*, 1862; courtesy of the University of Illinois Library.)

as the *Anne-Marie.* Some carried men sick with yellow fever and convalescents from the disease. The threat posed by the *Anne-Marie* was, as
every observer recognized, not that created by a casual arrival but by the
fleet of ships now engaged in the Caribbean trade.

A method was needed for dealing with this problem. Traditional or
full quarantine provided no reasonable solutions or acceptable practice.
Quarantine, if successfully enforced, simply prevented men, ships, and cargo
from entering a port for an often lengthy period of time. It could pose
a grave risk for persons who, trapped aboard a suspect vessel, had somehow been able to preserve their health during the crossing. Full quarantine
also brought commerce between a port and suspect foreign ports to a complete halt, entailing widespread and often large financial losses. A nation's
failure to impose quarantine in her ports could cause foreign nations to
refuse entrance of the offender's ships into their own ports.

After 1850, quarantine began to lose its original meaning, not just in
practice, where endless variations had always obtained, but also in officially sanctioned regulations. The participants at the first Sanitary Conference sought to define a flexible approach to the quarantine problem,
although without reaching agreement. The French degree of 1853 suggested
that the "length of quarantine will be the same for the ship, passengers,
and cargo," yet stated an important set of operational distinctions depending upon whether one faced the threat of plague, Asiatic cholera, or yellow
fever, and upon the circumstances under which each disease was encountered.[39] The length of quarantine of persons was made a function of the
ship's condition upon departure (her bill of health), her medical experience at sea, and her point of origin (Mediterranean or oceanic). In the worst
case, a quarantine of ten days was to be imposed on crewmen and passengers arriving from Turkey aboard a ship carrying the ominous *patente brute,*
that is, a foul bill of health. Cargo aboard all ships was allowed immediate
entry, except, again, that aboard an arrival from Turkey with *patente brute.*
Only arrivals from yellow-fever countries carrying a *patente brute* were
to be detained, a clear indication of the importationist foundation of yellow-
fever quarantine. There could be no yellow fever in France had there not
been yellow fever abroad and maritime contact with the infected region.
Such a notion, never forgotten, had been anathema to Chervin and the
early noncontagionist party.

Mélier continued this process of fine-tuning the French quarantine machinery. He sought to cut through previous hesitations and qualifications
and find measures that were at once feasible, effective, and specifically suited

39. Colin, "Quarantines," articles 50, 52, p. 65; Tardieu, "Sanitaire (Régime)," Annex
C, 3:318–319.

to his problem, the importation of yellow fever. Rather than hold men, ships, and cargo in sequestration for an indefinite period of time, he proposed and introduced the immediate disembarkation of men and goods and established a series of measures to be taken once disembarkation had begun. His method was embodied in a set of regulatory instructions that received ministerial approval on 16 August 1861, this being reconfirmed on the thirtieth and thereafter serving as the basis for French protective measures against the disease.[40] Mélier directed that all ships arriving from Havana or any other suspected yellow-fever port were to be diverted to an anchorage on the left bank of the Loire and refused entry into the roadstead or basin at Saint-Nazaire. In suspicious cases, when the ship carried an unclean bill of health or had suffered serious illness at sea, sanitary inquiry (*arraisonement*) by port authorities was to be conducted at a distance. The port physician then boarded the arrival and sought out actual or suspect cases of yellow fever. These persons were quickly transferred to a nearby hospital ship or hospital, there to be treated until recovery or death. All other persons not strictly needed to care for the vessel (crew members as well as passengers) were transferred to yet another ship. Here they were to remain for three to seven days. This period, the critical moment of the operation for passengers and crewmen, was one of observation and nothing else. Those who showed no illness at the close of the observation period were free to enter the country and go about their business unhindered; the sick were to be hospitalized. This routine assured the separation of the sick and the seemingly well, the latter receiving thereby additional protection from the disease.

To this point, no real risk had been taken. Opening the hatches and penetrating into the hold — where risk turned into outright peril — were prohibited until the most likely victims had been removed from the ship. Unloading then began; it was conducted very slowly, while the vessel still lay at anchor. Those few who conducted these operations would unavoidably expose themselves to some danger. The ship being cleaned and thoroughly ventilated, chlorine led the way into the hold. Cargo, ship's timbers, and decking were all well covered with a semifluid chlorine paste; step-by-step, as the process moved deeper into the hold, every object and structure

40. The text of these instructions was reproduced in Mélier, "Relation de la fièvre jaune survenue à Saint-Nazaire," pièce 19, pp. 185–186; an English translation appears in "Report by Dr. George Buchanan on the Outbreak of Yellow Fever at Swansea," *Parliamentary Papers* 33 (1866) [Reports from Commissioners. 17. Pollution of Rivers. Public Health; i.e., Eighth Report of the Medical Officer of the Privy Council, with Appendices, 1865]: 469–470. The translation is followed by commentary by John Simon (pp. 470–474). Michel Lévy, *Traité d'hygiène publique et privée*, 2 vols., 6th ed. (Paris: J. B. Baillière, 1879), 2:378–379, reports briefly on these developments.

was coated. The liquid flowed down over sugar barrels and the inner sides of the ship and in so doing disinfected all that it touched. Once in the bilge, it treated that cesspool and gave rise to vapors that then penetrated upwards into all parts of the vessel and its cargo. Not a step was to be taken without preparing the way with chlorine solution.

The cargo, now well chlorinated, was placed aboard lighters or barges and kept in the open air. The barges remained moored near the ship until movement was authorized by the port physician. Then, still in open air, the cargo moved on to Nantes. Transport by water kept human contact with the sugar to a minimum until thorough aeration had occurred. Although it had not been associated with any accidents, the railroad was distrusted because it entailed too much contact between cargo and susceptibles. The final operations on the ship consisted of cleaning and scraping the interior of the vessel and soaking it repeatedly with chlorine solution. The interior was then dried and whitewashed, a dilute chlorine solution being added to the whitewash. Upon inspection and approval by the port physician, the ship could be released to its owner.

To Mélier, traditional quarantine reflected both failure of nerve and inexcusable inattention to the lessons of science. Quarantine merely temporized; its program was inactivity. Mélier himself demanded action. The measures applied to the *Anne-Marie* and other ships offered a major modification of quarantine for yellow fever without eliminating it. That modification was the most important aspect of the matter. It revealed how knowledge and action might be combined, thus exhibiting the potential hygienic powers of the rising science of epidemiology.

This active mode informed Mélier's entire inquiry and it allowed him to state his claim for innovation.

> Instead of temporizing, the characteristic feature of the old quarantine, sanitary unloading offers immediate action. . . . There are two advantages to this: the first is to preserve public health more effectively and the second is to gain precious time, time whose value we appreciate today more than ever and which we must learn to conserve, whatever be the price.
>
> If I am not mistaken, the system of sanitary unloading, conducted for the first time in this manner at Saint-Nazaire, constitutes genuine progress in the provision of sanitary care. A few words summarize it all: *greater security and economizing of time.*[41]

Quarantine simply declared: keep them out for a set period of days. This reflected a hope that time alone would allow the disease to run its course among this isolated population and thus eliminate the threat of importa-

41. Mélier, "Relation de la fièvre jaune survenue à Saint-Nazaire," p. 64.

tion. Sanitary action stated: let them in but take great care in how their entrance is effected. To the new sanitarian, "them" referred to a set of sharply differentiated objects. Men and women might enter quickly, after a short period of observation; cargo could enter immediately, just as soon as provisions for secure sanitary discharge could be put into effect. The ship, too, could be sanitized but, because it was truly the infected party, it was to be kept in complete isolation until the necessary operations had been completed. There was no need for *sabordement* or other destructive intervention with regard to this valuable property. Mélier believed, quite rightly, that the overall "method" represented here, together with the implementation of that method, constituted the novelty of his work.[42] To be sure, his method was composed of familiar elements, but these elements and the ensemble they formed were now based upon facts taken from close observation and analysis of an exemplary epidemic of a specific disease. Here conclusions were not derived from general principles but from a meticulous local inquiry and keen attention to the epidemiological character of the disease of interest.

The Incubation Period

Sanitary unloading required attention to all that entered a port: ship, cargo, and human beings. The latter posed special questions. Some men and women were ill upon arrival, others were to all appearances healthy. The seriously ill could be readily identified and, if it were thought necessary, isolated. But what about the well? Did they pose a threat to themselves or to the community at large? How was one to deal with this possibility?

From time immemorial it has been recognized that disease is not communicated instantaneously. Between the moment of supposed contact and the appearance of sickness in a new victim, a certain, if indefinite, period of time must elapse. Around 1800 this general notion of a "latent" or, as it has become known, "incubation" period began to receive much clearer medical formulation. The incubation period was another of those features that contributed to the distinctness of each communicable disease. George Gregory in 1829 declared that "each particular contagion acknowledges a different law" in respect to the onset of symptoms after contact, and his conclusion only gained in strength over the following decades.[43]

It was, however, far easier to entertain the notion of an incubation pe-

42. Ibid., p. 65.
43. See H. K. Armenian and A. M. Lilienfeld, "Incubation Period of Disease," *Epidemiologic Reviews* 5 (1983): 1–15. Passage cited, p. 1.

riod than it was to establish accurately the length of such a period. In certain diseases, notably smallpox and rabies, which were accepted as being wholly contagious, it was possible to determine with considerable precision the moment of contact between sick and susceptible and thus to ascertain the length of the incubation period. The contagiousness of other and important diseases, however, remained in doubt; no such direct calculation was possible for typhoid or typhus fever, Asiatic cholera, the malarial fevers, or yellow fever. For the believer in contagion regarding one or another of these diseases, the issue was further complicated by the prevailing ignorance of the nature of the contact between the hypostatized pathogen and the potential victim.

Mélier needed a good estimate of the incubation period of yellow fever. Certainly the subject had received ample attention. Every imaginable period, from hours and days to weeks and months, had been suggested, although most commonly entertained was a relatively brief period of up to two weeks. The modified quarantine procedures embodied in Mélier's scheme of sanitary unloading made a new resolution of the matter essential. His program required a prescribed period of observation in a hospital-ship or a hospital; efficiency and humanity, as well as safety, demanded that this period be as brief as was consistent with hygienic efficacy.

Strong views were held regarding the incubation period, including Mélier's. Whatever one's notion of the cause of the disease was, an observer had to start with the declaration of sickness in an affected individual. Assuming that very early diagnosis was possible (and diagnosis of yellow fever at any stage but especially at onset was very difficult) a crucial reference point was established. One could now reason backwards in time to previous actual or potential contacts. But what was an authentic yellow-fever contact? The answer to this question depended upon how one viewed the etiology of the disease. The contagionist sought out person-to-person contact between the new yellow-fever victim and an earlier victim(s); Mélier, rather to his surprise, had done just this in the case of Alphonse Chaillon. The noncontagionist with equal ease connected one or usually several victims to peculiar miasmatic conditions; Mélier followed this course in explaining most cases of yellow fever at Saint-Nazaire.

Under the earlier noncontagionist interpretation of a yellow-fever epidemic, the notion of an incubation period could lose definition or even importance. Contact with a miasma, the latter itself sufficiently ill-circumscribed, was no doubt in order, but the critical questions of when and where contact was made could not be satisfactorily answered. A miasma ashore was a very general, not to say diffuse affair. Its limits could be established only by its effect, a relatively high incidence of disease. There were no other parameters, save perhaps the presence of an unwholesome smell and this, as the Gibraltar reports indicate, was neither always present nor perceived in the same manner by different observers.

Locating this miasma, or whatever be the causal agent, aboard a ship introduced an important new parameter. Under favorable circumstances, a ship's arrival was a datable event. Within the importationist interpretation of yellow fever, it was the crucial event in establishing a well-grounded estimate of the incubation period of the disease. The *Anne-Marie* constituted the indisputable *terminus a quo* at Saint-Nazaire. Infectious contact before the ship's arrival, whether person-to-person or by miasma, was obviously impossible. Moreover, although she had entered the basin on 25 July, the *Anne-Marie* was carrying convalescents but no sick individuals. She had begun unloading her cargo only on the twenty-seventh. Subsequent events suggested that the infective agent had lurked in the hold of the ship, contained there like a bomb ready to explode. The opening of the hatches and penetration into the hold by new susceptibles thus constituted the beginning of the spread of the disease. The twenty-seventh, therefore, was taken as the starting point for all contacts; 3 August, when unloading was completed, was accepted as the last possible contact date. Eloy, the supervising officer, fell ill on the second. Numerous others followed on the third through the sixth, and the last new case of a stricken stevedore declared itself on 11 August.

From these facts, Mélier concluded that the poison of yellow fever is *"a rapidly acting poison."* This followed from his opinion, with regard to this "capital question of incubation period," that, "given one or more individuals exposed to yellow fever, I feel I may declare and I do so declare that we should know very quickly what the [temporal limits] are. Thus, as I stated in my report, new cases appear beginning on the second day, most often on the third or fourth day and rarely on the fifth, sixth or seventh days. . . . It goes without saying that there is nothing absolute about these conclusions and that certain exceptions to them are not excluded."[44] Without a definite reference point, the mere announcement of a three- to seven-day incubation period had no meaning. The arrival of the *Anne-Marie*, together with the demonstration that yellow fever was an imported disease, provided just this reference point and thus constituted a sound foundation for reasoning on the question of the incubation period of yellow fever.

In the wide-ranging discussion of his report at the Academy of Medicine, Mélier faced a number of challenges, not least regarding the announced

44. Mélier, "Discussion sur la fièvre jaune," *Bulletin de l'Académie impériale de médecine* 28 (1862–1863): 994–995. This "Discussion," involving many participants and occupying several days, constituted a thorough review of Mélier's entire inquiry at Saint-Nazaire. It appears in the *Bulletin* thus: pp. 646–695; 834–891; 977–1039.

incubation period of yellow fever. In reply to his colleague, Jules Guérin, a stalwart of the yellow-fever debates since the 1830s and a bold and eclectic theoretician, Mélier hewed close to the facts. Guérin wanted an absolutely complete account of events aboard the *Anne-Marie* and in Saint-Nazaire, even if such an account should slide far into conjecture. Mélier knew that such an account was impossible. He was especially careful in regard to the question of the length of the incubation period of yellow fever, making the essential methodological point that in many and perhaps in most cases one cannot determine when exposure to the disease principle began. The best that could be done, and this only in some cases, was to determine with accuracy the date when exposure surely ended.[45] The stevedores aboard the *Anne-Marie* offered a case in point. Unloading was completed on 3 August, and the ship was isolated in the center of the basin on the fifth. Exposure of the stevedores was obviously most unlikely after the third and was quite impossible after the fifth. Did, then, contact between infectious agent and victim occur on the first day or the last, early in the period of exposure or late? Despite Guérin's urging, Mélier knew that he could not answer this question, and he did not. What could be concluded with assurance was that, in all cases in which the evidence was complete and the times of possible exposure and confirmed attack clearly stated, the incubation period was of short duration, a period of three to seven days. The date, 3 August, was evidently used to establish this period. An incubation period of three to seven days was therefore placed in the Regulatory Instructions of August, 1861; it served to confirm the provisions already stated in the Sanitary Decree of 1853.[46]

Obviously, not everyone was prepared to accept this period or related arguments. The experience of the *Anne-Marie* at sea seemed to raise a number of exciting alternative interpretations. All evidence indicated that she had not been a sick ship when she left Havana. None of her crew was then ill and she gave no signs of trouble to come. When yellow fever did appear on board, she had been long at sea; the first case of disease appeared on 1 July, seventeen days after leaving Havana on 13 June. Guérin thought he could explain this delay without great difficulty. The process of infection was, he believed, a gradual process, one analogous to fermentation in that increments of small magnitude could generate a major change. This led to the conclusion that the members of the crew, contrary to what had been stated, were infected when they boarded the vessel in Havana. Their condition then and for many days thereafter was not, however, acute.

45. Ibid., pp. 997–998.
46. Mélier, "Relation de la fièvre jaune survenue à Saint-Nazaire," pièce 19, Article 8, p. 185.

This was the "prodromic period" of the disease, a condition often proposed but which usually evaded the eye of even an experienced physician, not to mention a sailor or ship's captain. During the hot days of the passage through the Straits of Florida the ferment of yellow fever multiplied in the bodies of the infected crewmen. At the same time these ferments were escaping by means of "pulmonary and cutaneous emanations." Becoming now true "morbific germs," the real thing with regard to infection, they accumulated aboard the ship. Days later, they burst forth and this time overwhelmed their victims. All of this, Guérin averred, was "no hypothesis, but a fact of everyday observation," one always associated with "virulent and contagious diseases."[47]

Guérin's definition of fact was very different from that of other experts, including Mélier. The latter tended to scoff at Guérin's grander fancies, but he addressed carefully the conclusion made to follow from his colleague's analysis, namely, yellow fever may have an incubation period of seventeen days or more, or it may be only two days long, or perhaps any period between these limits. In fact, it might be pointless to contemplate an incubation "period" of any length for the disease. Mélier objected, and fairly so, that Guérin always selected what was possible, not what was likely or demonstrable, and that in making his selection he chose dates that assured a long incubation period.[48] Many facts favored a much shorter period. Still, one could not deny the events aboard the *Anne-Marie* herself. No active case of yellow fever had boarded the ship, yet precisely that disease and no other broke out a full seventeen days after all connection with an infected port and other human beings had been severed. Many another ship had experienced this same perplexing sequence of events, and a solution to the riddle was nowhere near to hand.[49]

Guérin's proposals might be answered but could not be refuted. The

47. Jules Guérin, "Discussion sur la fièvre jaune," *Bulletin de l'Académie impériale de médecine* 28 (1862–1863): 853.

48. Ibid.

49. Just what had caused the epidemic aboard the *Anne-Marie*? One can only speculate. It is highly improbable that all the afflicted crewmen had had exceptionally long incubation periods. Furthermore, if such an explanation is offered, the problem arises of where the infective agent (virus) resided upon arrival in Saint-Nazaire. One could argue that it traveled with the men, but then one would need to declare allegiance to the contagiousness of yellow fever and person-to-person transmission. More likely, the ship in Havana took aboard mosquitoes early in the (extrinsic) incubation period and these mosquitoes, at a later date — when they had become infective — attacked susceptible crew members, thereby passing the virus to man. Combining the broader limits of the extrinsic and intrinsic incubation periods permits the observed delay of seventeen to twenty-five days in the appearance of shipboard yellow fever. Mosquitoes could easily have survived until the ship reached France, infective until their death; other generations of mosquitoes might also have been involved.

answers varied. Jean Louis Poiseuille, for example, rejected a long incubation period for yellow fever. He explained events aboard the *Anne-Marie* by the fact or, rather, the claim that members of the crew had been "habituated" to the disease during their long visit in Havana.[50] But once Havana's atmosphere was left behind—and that portion that was carried away remained well isolated in the ship's tightly sealed hold—the crew "for seventeen days lived in a different environment. Their bodies must have changed and this change has caused them to lose the immunity that they enjoyed upon departure." The great heat of the passage through the Straits of Florida then caused the vitiated air in the hold to expand and it crept through the bulkheads separating hold and crew's quarters. An epidemic at sea inevitably ensued, beginning almost three weeks into the voyage. Poiseuille, whose personal acquaintance with yellow fever and its victims was nil, simply ignored the well-established fact that a bona fide case of yellow fever conferred lasting immunity. *Habituation,* or *acclimatization,* a widely accepted but ill-explained process, might thus be used to understand the epidemic at sea, but only at the price of implying that some form of protective immunity had been acquired and was then soon lost.[51]

Mélier ignored Poiseuille's suggestion just as he denied Guérin's hypothesis. His own explanation of the long-delayed outbreak of yellow fever aboard the *Anne-Marie* formed an integral part of his major conclusion drawn from the epidemic at large: the ship, not the men, had been infected upon departure from Havana. "As a general proposition," he noted,

> we may conclude that, when yellow fever has been contracted [by an individual] at the point of departure, three, four or five days at sea do not pass without it making itself evident. If its appearance is delayed beyond this period, you may be assured that the cause of the disease lies elsewhere, that it resides in the ship herself or in certain of the objects that she carries.[52]

Momentarily in accord with Guérin, Mélier tied this "cause" to the presence of ferments. "In my view . . . this doctrine of ferments and fermenta-

50. J. L. Poiseuille, "Discussion sur la fièvre jaune," *Bulletin de l'Académie impériale de médecine* 28 (1862–1863): 889.

51. Acclimatization referred to that seasoning process whereby newcomers to an unhealthy station experienced a long or short siege of ailments, some severe, and then emerged relatively resistant or immune to local hazards. The notion was usually applied to European experience in malarious regions, especially settlers in the Americas, and is met but rarely with reference to yellow fever. See Hirsch, *Handbook of Geographical and Historical Pathology* 1:346–348 (yellow fever), 243–247 (malaria). Also L. A. Bertillon, "Acclimatement, Acclimatation," *Dictionnaire encyclopédique des sciences médicales* 1:270–323; J. B. Fonssagrives, "Assuétude," ibid., 6:700–702.

52. Mélier, "Discussion sur la fièvre jaune," p. 1000.

tion explains the facts, especially those of the crossing; it offers a most satisfying interpretation of these facts, one to which I give my full allegiance." But immediately the important difference between the two interpretations revealed itself. The notion of ferments, Mélier explained,

> allows us to understand how the [causal] principle of the disease—whether this principle be plant or animal, cryptogam or infusorian is unimportant— having come aboard a ship, persists there, increases [in number] and develops [its potentialities]. It does this in a manner different from inert [nonliving] bodies. It acts, so all appearances suggest, in the same way that bodies endowed with a modicum of life act; it gives birth to the infection. It is in this manner, or by some other unknown operation related to chemical reactions, that this infection can be present and in fact probably is present. And all of this can occur without there being necessarily present, as part of the explanation, sick human beings.[53]

This statement, although a truly wondrous expression of the manifold etiological possibilities that had become available in the 1860s, could not assure the resolution of the matter of the length of the incubation period of yellow fever.

To Mélier, Guérin's hypothesis suggested at best the independent existence of a causal ferment; to Guérin, that hypothesis meant that a human victim was always required in order to provide a host for the infective agent. Neither observer possessed any tangible evidence regarding the behavior of the supposed infective agent, just as there was no direct evidence that such an agent even existed. Obviously, both interpreters were capable of reaching well beyond the seeming facts of the matter and finding themselves lost in sheer speculation. However, the relationship proposed between a putative infective agent of yellow fever and the presence or absence of sick individuals does bring up the questions then being raised by the incipient germ theory of disease; these will be the subject of the following chapter.

The disagreements expressed in the discussion of Mélier's report at the Academy of Medicine in 1863, however, pertained to matters of general scientific interest. But Mélier realized that the practical domain must be the ultimate consideration in deciding how best to mount a hygienic defense against the importation of yellow fever. The solution was to require the sanitary unloading of ships and men. "Let us not conclude," he observed,

> that we have here [in the incubation period] a matter of no importance, one of simple scientific curiosity. . . . I know of no question more important in

53. Ibid., p. 1011.

the study of yellow fever and its connection to sanitary activity. On this matter, on the solution that we adopt to this problem, depends our entire system
of preventive measures.

   If we admit, as I believe we should, that the incubation period is short,
then a few days' observation [of incoming persons] is sufficient. If, to the contrary, we suppose that the incubation period is long, ten or twenty, even thirty,
forty or more days, as M. Guérin in effect does suppose by his way of reasoning, we inevitably lapse into the old ways of a long quarantine. Such quarantines are today really beyond our administrative capabilities. Moreover, [if
they were imposed] they would render vain and illusory the rapidity of [mod-
ern] navigation and would ruin commerce.[54]

Thirty-five years earlier Chervin and his allies had pronounced yellow fever
to be noncontagious. Armed with this conclusion, they had sought loudly
and successfully to reduce or eliminate quarantine for this disease. What
were already inadequate and ill-enforced protective measures largely became no measures at all. Mélier was convinced that yellow fever was an
imported disease and that it might occasionally become, as the Chaillon
affair disclosed, a contagious disease. He therefore demanded and obtained
the reimposition of control measures for yellow fever. But, like Chervin
and most sanitarians of the epoch, he, too, had a nice sense of the pecu-
niary importance of international trade and of the seemingly inexorable
demands of the transportation revolution then underway. Regularity and
speed of transport were important matters in a nation's economic life. They
were not to be tampered with in a casual or doctrinaire manner. But public
health was also of major national interest and its protection a responsibility of any enlightened administration. Modified quarantine incorporat-
ing a major epidemiological conclusion, the short incubation period of
yellow fever, was a response that was held to satisfy both demands.

After the *Anne-Marie*

   Mélier's preliminary inquiries led quickly to the Regulatory Instructions of 16 August 1861. These instructions were immediately applied to
all ships from suspect ports that made Saint-Nazaire their destination. By
the twentieth of August, the hulk *Alcibiade,* capable of holding some forty
persons requiring observation, was in place on the new quarantine grounds
at Mindin across the Loire; a few days later the *Penelope,* devoted to hospital service, joined her. Mélier's instructions were followed to the letter
over the next four weeks, that is, during the remainder of what was thought
to be the yellow-fever season at this high latitude. What effect had these
measures on yellow fever in the town of Saint-Nazaire?

54. Ibid., pp. 1003–1004.

Of the fourteen ships that entered the Loire from Havana between the arrival of the *Anne-Marie* (25 July) and the twentieth of September, five had carried crew members who died of yellow fever during the crossing or after arrival. Another ship reported that several men had been sick in Havana, but no deaths occurred among them. Obviously, the Saint-Nazaire sugar fleet was an infected fleet and its potential for causing trouble in metropolitan France was not small. Yet, with one exception, nothing happened. As of 20 September, the port physician reported, "twelve ships have been unloaded and sanitized, two others are now completing these operations and, while all this work was being done, only one case of infection has occurred."[55]

That case was a singular one and seemed to prove beyond any doubt the truth of Mélier's contention that the ship itself was infected. The *Alphonse-Nicolas-Cézard* reached Saint-Nazaire from Havana on 16 August.[56] Two crew members were ill with yellow fever upon arrival and one subsequently died. Unloading began on 26 August; only three days later another yellow-fever victim appeared. Taken ill on the twenty-ninth, François-Marie Gennissel died on 5 September, the unique case of yellow fever ashore in the epidemic of 1861 that had no connection with the *Anne-Marie*. Gennissel was a laborer engaged in unloading and cleaning the *Alphonse-Nicolas-Cézard* and had been formally instructed to abide by the new rules governing access to the ship. By the time that unloading was begun, Mélier's Regulatory Instructions were in place and governed every step of the procedure. In Gennissel's case, these precautions were observed, yet a metropolitan susceptible had been stricken. Were the precautions therefore invalid?

Close inquiry revealed that Gennissel and his fellow workers had worked with great haste and had not conducted the disinfection operations with required thoroughness. As they reached ever lower in the ship's hold and neared the bilge (and thus the end of their onerous work) they paid insufficient heed to the massive chlorination required there of the water, debris, and packing materials (mostly broken branches) that crowded this deepest and, as everyone believed, most dangerous part of the ship. Here if anywhere the deadly miasma was to be found. Gennissel's death was of his own making and his fellows were fortunate to escape. The new sanitary regulations might be evaded, but they had not been called into question. The sickness and death of Gennissel was due to an infected ship and that, if not a laborer's foolish behavior, was a remediable matter.

These events closed the epidemic of yellow fever at Saint-Nazaire. Gen-

---

55. Mélier, quoting the port physician, Dr. Gestin, "Relation de la fièvre jaune survenue à Saint-Nazaire," p. 178. See also the *tableau*, p. 173.

56. Ibid., pp. 179–185, 56–57.

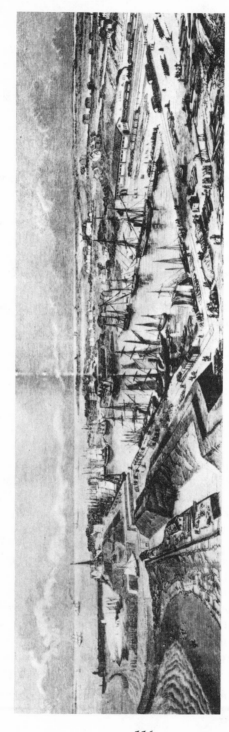

The port of Saint-Nazaire, 1857. This superb view, looking to the southwest, shows the construction of the tidal basin and connecting railroad lines (the main station would be constructed near the freight depot on the extreme right). In the upper left appears the old landing stage of the fishing village; to the right the full sweep of the new town. Virtually everything seen in this lithograph, except the main body of the tidal basin itself, was destroyed in the Second World War. (Gaston Le Floc'h and Fernand Guériff, *Saint-Nazaire* [Loire-Atlantique, 44] [Colmar-Ingersheim: Editions S.A.E.P., 1974], pp. 2–3.)

nissel was the last person ashore to take ill from the disease and the last person to die from it. Surveillance begun, however, was surveillance continued. Published in 1863, Mélier's report included data on the sanitary practice and experience of Saint-Nazaire in 1862 and data on the same year for the much more active ports of Marseilles and Toulon. Dozens of ships from suspect areas reached these several ports bearing unclean bills of health. Several ships had had aboard cases of yellow fever in their respective ports of departure (Havana, Matanzas, Trinidad, Rio de Janeiro, Vera Cruz), and others had seen the disease develop while at sea.[57] No sick or convalescents entered the Mediterranean ports in 1862, and only routine but careful execution of sanitary unloading was performed. The same operations were conducted at Saint-Nazaire where ten sugar ships bearing *patentes brutes* from Vera Cruz and Havana arrived. All were given close attention, including sanitary discharge of cargo and brief observation of crew members. Only one, however, the *Albert* from Havana, had had serious problems with yellow fever in the Cuban capital, at sea and upon arrival. Severe measures were taken with her. Aboard the seven passenger liners that arrived from Mexico (these belonging to the famous Compagnie Générale de Transport, newly founded and operating from Saint-Nazaire) no case of yellow fever had declared itself at any time.

From none of these ships did yellow fever move ashore. Like 1861, 1862 was a bad yellow-fever year in Havana, and communications with that port and others in the region were again numerous. The usual anxiety in the European ports proved, however, unfounded. Mélier believed that his sanitary measures were responsible for limiting the spread of the disease to contacts with the *Anne-Marie* and to Gennissel aboard the *Alphonse-Nicolas-Cézard*. He thought, too, that these measures, if properly enforced, would henceforth protect all Europe from similar invasions. To be sure, other and equally likely explanations for the safety of Saint-Nazaire can be proposed. From a twentieth-century perspective, the key fact is that an infective mosquito and a susceptible human being did not come together. Why this happened has many possible explanations, ranging from a lack of susceptibles or the occurrence of the disease in unrecognized subacute form, to interruption of the chain of transmission at sea, or environmental conditions (especially temperature) unfavorable to mosquitoes at the port of arrival. It is also possible that massive chlorination and the resulting fumes purged the offending ships of mosquitoes. There is today no way to sort through these or other possible explanations and resolve the question.

57. For arrivals in Saint-Nazaire in 1862, ibid., pp. 198–199; for those in Mediterranean ports in the same year, ibid., pp. 210–215.

The epidemic of 1861 constituted the one and only serious outbreak of yellow fever to affect the French homeland. With regard to the development of epidemiological methods, how the investigation of the epidemic was conducted was far more important than the events themselves. In contrast to the situation encountered in previous European outbreaks of the disease, the "facts" at Saint-Nazaire were, as Mélier himself had stated, "not numerous and they were as clear as they could be." Just here was his advantage, and it was his peculiar genius to appreciate the opportunity set before him. Proud of his accomplishment, he insisted that this epidemic was to be "considered a type or specimen against which we may compare analogous facts and which gives us the means by which to evaluate these new facts."[58] The epidemic at Saint-Nazaire may be viewed as an exemplary epidemic, one that allowed epidemiologists to discover and define essential general parameters of epidemic yellow fever, thus establishing a solid and suggestive basis for further investigation.[59]

By no means had Mélier's inquiry answered all questions regarding the transmission of the disease. Some issues, many noted above, passed unnoticed, and others received only brief consideration. The etiological question, however, was not among these. Its importance was recognized and its dimensions assayed, even though such consideration led only to frustration. Neither Mélier nor his contemporaries made much progress when, with hopeful but doomed speculation, they attempted to augment their understanding of the epidemiology of yellow fever with an elucidation of the cause of the disease.

58. Mélier, "Discussion sur la fièvre jaune," 91.
59. See L. G. Stevenson, "A Pox on the Illeum: Typhoid Fever among the Exanthemata," *Bulletin of the History of Medicine* 51 (1977): 496–505; idem, "Exemplary Disease: The Typhoid Pattern," *Journal of the History of Medicine* 37 (1982): 159–181. As has been seen, critical to Mélier's interpretation was the conclusion that yellow fever possessed its own epidemiological character and that sanitary measures can be effective only if designed to fit this character. With the return of Asiatic cholera in 1865–1866, the French government applied Mélier's lesson to efforts to counteract the new scourge. Modified quarantine was employed and all measures were reconsidered and then tailored to fit the perceived epidemiological character of cholera. See Fauvel, *Le choléra*, pp. 41–72, 421–483. These measures were imposed by an Imperial decree of 23 June 1866: Lévy, *Traité d'hygiène publique et privée* 2:379–380.

5

Saint-Nazaire: Etiology

THIS BRIEF CHAPTER deals with confusion. It is time to address directly the problem of disease causation as it was understood in the 1860s and with reference to yellow fever. The familiar themes of contagion and noncontagion continued to dominate the etiological landscape, although intimations of the germ theory of disease were already present. François Mélier at Saint-Nazaire conducted a fundamentally epidemiological investigation, but he obviously did not fail to notice closely related causal questions. His problem, and that of all others who explored these questions, was that the much sought-after causal agent of yellow fever remained unknown. A specific causal entity was much discussed and pursued but never captured. Neither for the first nor the last time, a direct approach to the cause of yellow fever offered only disappointment.

Two decades later, the germ theory of disease began to revolutionize understanding of the character and transmission of communicable disease. The germ theory coordinated a series of fundamental discoveries relating specific microbes to specific diseases. It also set forth a programmatic position regarding the causation of communicable disease and stated rules for demonstrating such a causal connection. The germ theory gradually assumed its mature outline in the years between 1865 and 1885, a creation of many investigators working in several lands. The theory emerged from a multitude of seemingly disparate interests: fermentation and the chemical processes of life, parasitism, bacterial taxonomy, field study of epidemic disease, microscopy, alternation of generations, and clinical medicine and surgery. The core of the germ theory of disease was disease causation.

Louis Pasteur, a chief author of the germ theory, made this abundantly clear in one of his first general pronouncements (1878) regarding the new doctrine.

> At the very beginning of our researches — and no sooner do we begin the latter than a new world reveals itself — what must be our most insistent demand? It is this: we seek absolute proof that there exist transmissible, contagious, infectious diseases the cause of each of which resides essentially and uniquely in the presence of microscopic organisms. We want to demonstrate that, for

a certain number of diseases, we must forever abandon the notion of spontaneous virulence, the idea of an infectious contagion [or] element that arises suddenly in the body of man or animals and serves as the origin of diseases which then spread further, all the while preserving their specific identity. All of these ideas are fatal to medical progress, having given rise to such gratuitous hypotheses as spontaneous generation, albuminoid ferments, hemiorganisms, archebiosis and a host of other conceptions that lack even the most rudimentary observational basis.[1]

Pasteur's remarks described a research program, one already in motion, and informed the medical world that consideration of communicable disease must emphasize the etiological question. To many, the new notion of disease causation also provided the long-sought theoretical foundation for public-health activity. Friedrich Löffler, the student of another founder of the germ theory, Robert Koch, and an innovative microbiologist in his own right, observed bluntly that public hygiene "must thank bacteriology for the scientific establishment of those facts by means of which the application of effective prophylaxis is alone made possible."[2] Implicit in this claim was the ungenerous thought that all hygienic activity undertaken prior to the germ theory had been based on insecure and probably erroneous foundations and therefore was certainly of limited efficacy.

But the public health official before 1880 could work with the minimal proposition that there would be no threat of an epidemic or even an isolated case of a particular communicable disease without a definite yet unknown cause. The converse proposition, however, soon came to generate more complex problems. If, on the germ theory, one granted the entrance of a microorganismic cause into a community, there immediately arose the obscurities surrounding the interacting biological dynamics of virulence, resistance, and immunity. The mere presence of a microbe did not necessitate the appearance of disease. In dealing with this issue, first brought to the fore after 1880 by Pasteur's study of rabies, essentially new domains of medical science and biology were created. The investigation of yellow fever, however, played no part in these developments until the twentieth century.

The essential and curious point regarding the study of the cause or causes of yellow fever in the later nineteenth century, the so-called golden age of bacteriology, was that emphasis had necessarily to be placed on matters epidemiological and not etiological. Not unexpectedly, there was keen

---

1. Louis Pasteur et al., "La théorie des germes et ses applications à la médecine et à la chirurgie," *Comptes rendus des séances de l'Académie des sciences* 86 (1878): 1041.

2. Friedrich Löffler, *Vorlesungen über die geschichtliche Entwicklung der Lehre von den Bacterien* (Leipzig: F. C. W. Vogel, 1887), p. v.

interest in and much experimental investigation of the various possible bacterial agents that could be supposed to cause the disease. These efforts afforded, however, an independent lesson in frustration, for no specific bacterium could be assigned to yellow fever and the causal question was not answered.[3] Only after 1900 did this depressing situation begin to change.

Into the 1870s, yellow fever was understood in terms of the traditional interpretive categories, contagion and noncontagion. Each had many times been discredited and each often restored to favor. Both drew their support from, or suffered the challenge of, the facts of transmission. That a distinct causal agent of yellow fever acutally existed was in little dispute after 1850. But the fact that it was referred to, almost indifferently, as a principle of infection, an infective agent, an unknown cause, or, most simply and unambiguously, the unknown, reveals that the inquirer had very little to reason upon save his conviction. Both contagionist and noncontagionist used this language. The truth was that the unknown was the unknowable, and the problem of yellow fever had to be approached on another course. This course was set largely by epidemiology and it directed mind and eye to temporal relations, person-to-person contacts, internal factors such as local sanitary and climatic conditions, and external factors such as inbound ships from tropical ports.

It will soon become evident that Mélier's reflections on the causal agent of yellow fever proved nothing and opened up no new paths for exploration. But they were an integral part of the investigation of yellow fever at Saint-Nazaire and they offer, together with contemporary expressions of opinion, an insight into etiological thinking just before the announcement of the germ theory of disease. In this case these reflections concern a disease about which the latter theory would make no reliable comment for another seventy years.

An Unknown Causal Agent

How better to test one's etiological intuitions than by analyzing a well-described epidemic? Nicolas Chervin, a master of the art, had explored numerous local outbreaks in his quest for support for the noncontagionist interpretation of yellow fever. The great epidemics at Barcelona and Gibraltar had offered an invitation to virtually all interested parties to find the key, the central causal key, to this terrifying scourge. A small epidemic offered many attractions, too.

3. See Margaret Warner, "Hunting the Yellow Fever Germ: The Principle and Practice of Etiological Proof in Late Nineteenth-Century America," *Bulletin of the History of Medicine* 59 (1985): 361–382.

At Saint-Nazaire, for example, Mélier found numerous interesting facts. He also felt obliged to renounce the agnostic stance of his predecessors, the three French commissioners who had investigated the Gibraltar epidemic. Discussion, he noted, produces insight, or so they say. Perhaps it

> would have done so, had these illustrious observers [Chervin, Pierre Charles Alexandre Louis, and Armand Trousseau], after having studied the facts with such care, thought it necessary to interpret those same facts. Unhappily, there was little agreement amongst these observers; they themselves admitted it. They preferred to abstain from discussion and it was probably better that they did so. Besides, their orders read: *We ask of you facts and no opinions.* Finding myself in a different situation and having another mission, I shall try by means of reflection and by relating the facts one to another to venture some conclusions. Indeed, I consider it my duty to do so.[4]

Polite words, perhaps, and necessary. Louis was then living in retirement outside Paris, but Trousseau, at the peak of his career, listened to Mélier's presentation before the Academy of Medicine and joined the ensuing discussion. Since the 1820s the Academy had been the seat of acrimonious and inconclusive debates over rival etiological explanations of yellow fever and other communicable diseases. Yet even academicians grow weary of such struggles, and by the 1850s the use of terms such as *contagionism* and *noncontagionism* was meeting with distinctly less favor.[5] Mélier tried to avoid this language but often without success.

What, he asked, is the agent of infection and how does it come aboard and leave a ship? What is the connection between this agent and the atmosphere? Can the causal agent of the disease be transferred from person to person? In spite of patent unease, Mélier answered these questions and produced the outline of a disease theory, one that offered virtually no original elements. Being empirically well-founded, however, and receiving the Academy's formal approbation, it did shatter major components of Chervin's intellectual legacy. It thereby authorized the officially sanctioned reimposition of sanitary control over yellow fever and destroyed the primary practical application of Chervin's ideas.

4. François Mélier, "Relation de la fièvre jaune survenue à Saint-Nazaire en 1861," *Mémoires de l'Académie impériale de médecine* 26 (1863): 67.

5. In 1868 Auguste Fauvel called for rejection of further use of the term "contagion," this word being but an invitation to "logomachy," and insisted that henceforth only "transmission" constitute the subject-matter of the student of communicable disease. See his *Le choléra. Etiologie et prophylaxie* (Paris: J. B. Baillière, 1868), pp. 22–32. To others, however, the return of contagionist language and concepts seemed a great advance on the chaos of the era of P. J. B. Broussais and Nicolas Chervin: Charles Anglada, *Traité de la contagion,* 2 vols. (Paris: J. B. Baillière, 1853), 2:46.

Mélier kept no secrets. "What is this infection" that causes yellow fever, he asked, and "what is the poison that produces it? Nothing, certainly, would be more interesting for us to know. Unhappily, we are totally ignorant in these matters and I, for my part, have nothing whatsoever that I can use to clarify the problem."[6] With regard to some ships, those infested with typhus fever, for example, one might hypothesize that the severe crowding of men concentrates the maleficent miasma exhaled by each infected person. The spread of the disease results from this concentration. But this well-worn hypothesis, Mélier realized, held no meaning for the *Anne-Marie*. She carried sugar—vegetable, not animal, matter, and this remained in excellent condition throughout the entire voyage. Furthermore, she was not a crowded ship.

But a new hypothesis had just been announced. Its potential for explaining events aboard, of all things, a ship carrying sugar can easily be imagined. We are all now aware, Mélier noted, of recent studies of fermentation, particularly those that

> M. Pasteur has pursued so vigorously. In reading of this work, one is led almost in spite of oneself to ask if unfortunate events like those that we have just witnessed [in Saint-Nazaire] are not related to this important phenomenon. Fermentation, a process so different from ordinary chemical reactions, seems to belong as much to physiology as to chemistry, for it appears that in fermentation some kind of living entity [*une sorte de vie*] is always present.[7]

In 1863, however, neither Mélier nor his colleagues knew how to exploit this promising suggestion, least of all how to apply it to understanding the transmission of yellow fever.

Pasteur's experimental work seemed, nonetheless, to corroborate a familiar enough opinion, namely, communicable diseases and perhaps diseases in general each possessed a specific, even living, causal agent. Mélier regarded this conclusion to be essential to the whole notion of the importation of infectious disease.

> Whatever opinion we may hold regarding the nature of the principle that produces yellow fever, whether it be a miasma or a germ, a cryptogam or an infusorian, one thing seems certain. Once taken, we may say *loaded*, aboard a ship at point of departure, this principle is preserved therein and during the crossing probably also develops its potentialities and becomes much concentrated. As long as it is contained, it remains more or less latent and without effect. Its presence may sometimes be revealed during the passage, but

6. Mélier, "Relation de la fièvre jaune survenue à Saint-Nazaire," p. 74.
7. Ibid., p. 75.

it becomes immediately evident at the moment of arrival when the unloading of the ship sets it at liberty. Now, in the foregoing is contained all that we know regarding the cause of new cases; the nature of this cause altogether escapes us.[8]

Although of a nature unknown, such a cause could not be denied to exist.

So seemingly obvious a conclusion provokes a digression. Mélier concluded that what was imported was the cause of a disease, not the disease itself. This accorded well with the growing reductionist view of communicable disease, a view which tended to separate, at least analytically, cause (unknown agent or specific microbe) and effect (the diseased individual).[9] There was great power in this approach and there were also serious limitations.

On the one hand, the recognition of a distinct cause, such as a microbe, recommended the use of special prophylactic measures. Experience revealed that these measures — segregation of passengers; disinfection of goods, ship, clothing, or housing; purification of water supplies; and sanitary disposal of human and other wastes — could halt the spread of an epidemic or even prevent the entrance of disease, when properly conceived and systematically applied. This action was conducted on a purely external basis, that is, it proceeded effectively even when one had no idea of how the pathogen worked its harmful effect within the host. One needed only an understanding of how the unknown agent was transmitted from one point to another.

On the other hand, the strictly sanitary approach could divert attention from the disease process. In some cases, sanitarians of the bacteriological era saw fit to do without even the basic notion of a causal germ or germs. Certainly, study of the pathological processes induced by specific microbes posed profound technical and conceptual problems, and these were not easily or quickly overcome. Yet here, too, effective preventive measures could be devised, if only for a limited array of diseases. Pasteur and his school and, soon thereafter, Emil von Behring and his collaborators discovered the efficacy of artificial immunization (rabies) and serotherapy (tetanus and diphtheria antitoxins).[10] These were measures that

8. Ibid.

9. See Knud Faber, *Nosography. The Evolution of Clinical Medicine in Modern Times*, 2d ed. (New York: P. B. Hoeber, 1930), pp. 95–111.

10. See L. G. Stevenson, "Science Down the Drain: On the Hostility of Certain Sanitarians to Animal Experimentation, Bacteriology and Immunology," *Bulletin of the History of Medicine* 29 (1955): 1–29; W. H. Bulloch, *The History of Bacteriology* (London: Oxford University Press, 1960), pp. 241–283; Allan Chase, *Magic Shots. A Human and Scientific Account of the Long and Continuing Struggle to Eradicate Infectious Diseases by Vaccination*

served both public hygiene and the treatment of individuals. Once perfected and extended, and augmented by similar procedures applicable to other diseases (including artificial immunization against yellow fever, introduced in 1932), they became indispensable tools in every comprehensive program of disease control or eradication.

Until the 1880s, however, these weapons from the laboratory were unknown. In the previous decade, the notion of the microbial origin of communicable disease had itself remained no more than a suggestion. And for yellow fever, once again, no satisfying explanation of causation was offered during the nineteenth century, by the germ theory of disease or by any other proposal. This only reaffirms a point often stated earlier: epidemiology, not etiology, stands at the heart of the study of yellow fever at mid-nineteenth century and long after. In the case of many diseases, the germ theory did transform medical understanding; in fact, a new view of the causation of a disease could revolutionize one's conception of the epidemiology of that disease.[11] But even in the case of an important communicable disease such as Asiatic cholera, where laboratory culture of the microorganism played a decisive part in elucidating the disease cycle, there were critical moments when experimental measures failed and field studies and case-tracing were called upon to complete one's understanding. Robert Koch, for example, whose bacteriological discoveries form the core of the germ theory of disease, was an accomplished epidemiologist.[12]

The observer of the 1860s knew only that the causal question still defied resolution. Rather, he knew the traditional answers to this question and knew their shortcomings, too; yet he did not hesitate to offer these answers afresh if it seemed that a thorough ventilation of the problem was in order. Some observers entertained new suspicions such as those spoken by Mélier regarding the supposed cryptogamic or infusorial agent apparently at work in Saint-Nazaire; for this suggestion there was no proof of

---

(New York: William Morrow, 1982), pp. 114–190. Also A. P. Waterson and Lise Wilkinson, *An Introduction to the History of Virology* (Cambridge: Cambridge University Press, 1978).

11. See C. T. Gregg, *Plague. An Ancient Disease in the Twentieth Century*, rev. ed. (Albuquerque: University of New Mexico Press, 1985), pp. 129–231; René Dubos and Jean Dubos, *The White Plague. Tuberculosis, Man and Society* (Boston: Little, Brown, 1952), pp. 154–228.

12. The cholera vibrio could not be communicated to an experimental animal; it was therefore necessary to discover in the community points of contact between humans and the microbe in order to complete the demonstration of the pathogenic role of the vibrio. See Robert Koch's contributions to the two Berlin cholera conferences: "Erste Konferenz zur Erörterung der Cholerafrage am 26. Juli 1884 in Berlin," in *Robert Koch (1843–1910), Bakteriologe, Tuberkuloseforscher, Hygieniker. Ausgewählte Texte*, Sudhoffs Klassiker der Medizin. N.F. 2, edited with an Introduction by Paul Steinbrück and Achim Thom (Leipzig: J. A. Barth, 1982), pp. 141–170; "Conferenz zur Erörterung der Cholera-frage (Zweites Jahr)," *Deutsche medicinische Wochenschrift* 11, no. 37A (1885): 1–60.

any kind. In the end, discussion of the origin of yellow fever at Saint-Nazaire revolved about atmospheric causation and its modalities. Thus had such discussions run for at least sixty years.

A reasonable place to look for an answer to the causal question was the point of narrowest connection, namely, a ship leaving from or arriving at a sickly or healthy port. Mélier understood that it was vain to attempt to determine how the causal agent had boarded a ship in the harbor at Havana. It could have come aboard with corrupted water supplies or unclean wood and packing materials. It could also have arrived as a *"miasma-impregnated air."* However, because "no research has ever been conducted on this problem," there was no way to resolve the question.[13]

More obvious was the way in which the agent had left the vessel. The causal principle either attacked susceptibles who boarded the ship and were struck down or it affected individuals who carried the agent away with them, this being the only possible explanation of the illness of Alphonse Chaillon; the agent also could move away with the prevailing wind. Cargo and other effects from the ship did not convey the principle to new parties.

Mélier discussed the etiological question only within the relatively narrow framework set by events at Saint-Nazaire. His contemporaries addressed this question in a more general manner. Jean-Baptiste Fonssagrives, for example, discussed the etiology of yellow fever at length. Professor of medicine and hygiene in the naval medical school in Brest and then at the University of Montpellier, Fonssagrives had traveled widely in tropical areas. He knew yellow fever firsthand and knew it well. "The origin of a contagion," he declared in his *Traité d'hygiène navale* (1856), "is unknown, but reasoning indicates that it can be produced only by spontaneous generation or by the metamorphosis of an infection." Prudently, he did not elucidate the process of spontaneous generation, but he thought a metamorphosis could be "easily explained."[14] Infection itself was the product of the vitiation of the air in a particular locality. Fonssagrives added the further and familiar hypothesis that, given suitable conditions, the infectious agent could then be transformed into a contagious agent. This explained how or, better, simply stated that an infectious, that is, noncontagious, disease could evolve into a contagious disease. Here was another expression of contingent contagionism. But contagion, Fonssagrives continued, was the more powerful disease agent. It was a truly "pathological" poison and stronger than the merely "chemical" poison of atmospheric infection, that is, the former worked its influence deep within the body tissues, causing extensive and severe damage.

13. Mélier, "Relation de la fièvre jaune survenue à Saint-Nazaire," p. 75.
14. J. B. Fonssagrives, *Traité d'hygiène navale* (Paris: J. B. Baillière, 1856), p. 214.

These reflections were, as usual, a combination of conjectural pathology and an extrapolation from the conditions under which particular diseases appeared to be contracted. Fonssagrives enjoyed no privileged access to the secrets of yellow-fever causation, but that did not hinder his presentation of several etiological dicta designed to resolve prevailing uncertainties.

> Contagion seems to be transmitted *preferentially* by material connection (contact or humors); infection is transmitted *preferentially* by aerial dissemination. Sometimes, however, contagion moves through the air (smallpox) and sometimes infection is transmitted by material contact (putrid injections, fouled water).[15]

A physical connection between agent and victim was obviously a feature common to both etiological doctrines. Equally obvious was the fact that mode of transmission provided no reliable criterion for distinguishing between the rival interpretations. Both contagion and infection were contingent, the behavior of each evidently due to factors other than the carrier or carriers that moved the different disease principles.

This was not a promising beginning. The argument remained uncertain. Fonssagrives observed that "contagion invaded victims one after another and in a sequence that generally can be observed; infection, in contrast, strikes immediately and simultaneously the greatest number of persons who are exposed to its action." Diseases designated contagious, including smallpox, syphilis, and plague, thus advanced person-by-person through a community. Often enough the outbreak was the result of the arrival in the community of an identifiable diseased individual or individuals. Infectious diseases, and Fonssagrives placed yellow fever in this group, attacked suddenly and affected whole communities. For these diseases usually no specific external contact or means of importation could be identified. His next proposition expressed long-established wisdom.

> The propagation of contagion is independent of any atmospheric influence; communication becomes increasingly probable as moribund and healthy bodies near one another. The propagation of infection, in contrast, is dependent upon local conditions (wind, climate, temperature) which accelerate or delay its spread.

This statement nicely contradicts the qualifications announced in the earlier proposition. It points up again the dilemma that Fonssagrives — and Mélier and all other observers — faced. When studied closely, the move-

---

15. This and the following several propositions of Fonssagrives's, ibid., pp. 214–215.

ment of yellow fever exhibited both contagious and infectious (noncontagious) properties, the former being exhibited occasionally and the latter being the usual rule.

This raised a further problem: "contagion generally attacks an individual only once, but infections do not arm the organism against a new attack." By the 1850s, however, medical opinion recognized that an attack of yellow fever commonly conferred lasting immunity upon the victim.[16] This meant that yellow fever must be a contagious disease. One had to balance this conclusion, however, against the claims of the preceding propositions, namely, that yellow fever is essentially an infectious disease.

Lastly, Fonssagrives pointed out that "contagion can act over considerable [geographical] distances, being transported far from its point of departure; infection does not exert an effect beyond a limited range." Given the fact that yellow fever seemed to haunt coastal regions and only rarely moved inland — not even into such propitious havens as marshes and crowded, filthy towns and cities — this proposition asserted anew the infectious character of the disease.

It was not easy for Fonssagrives's contemporaries to build a coherent view of epidemic yellow fever upon such propositions and reasoning. It is no easier for the historian to do so but he, happily, has not this responsibility. The physician of the 1860s, anxious observer of the accelerating contact between Europe and tropical lands, was much less relaxed.

Fonssagrives had seriously hoped, and attempted, to resolve the yellow-fever problem. His approach was comprehensive and cautious but his success was slight. He was not alone. Another astute observer of tropical diseases attempted to cut through all of this obscurity and contradiction; his weapon was largely bold resolve. Auguste Frédéric Dutroulau had spent many years in the French Antilles studying the diseases of the region before returning to Brest as chief naval physician in that important military port. He, too, published an important work on exotic diseases. With regard to yellow fever, he announced, "I believe that [it] has as its essential and original cause an infection that is peculiar to certain maritime localities, a specific miasma. Its general and secondary cause is the climate of the hot countries. . . . In order to avoid any preconception in this matter, it is best to avoid that inappropriate word, contagion, as a description of

16. Opinion regarding the durability of acquired immunity remained unsettled. G. M. Sternberg in 1903 observed: "Immunity [in yellow fever] is acquired by suffering an attack of the disease; this acquired immunity is not, however, absolute. Second attacks no doubt occasionally occur, although this has been denied by some authors." *Infection and Immunity with Special Reference to the Prevention of Infectious Diseases* (New York: G. P. Putnam, 1903), p. 260. Also Andrew Davidson, "Yellow Fever," in *A System of Medicine*, 15 vols., ed. T. C. Allbutt (New York: Macmillan, 1898), 3:394.

how the disease is propagated; what is really involved is an infection." Further consideration, however, led him to enter a necessary and not unexpected qualification: infection can "arise from sick men as well as from local conditions." The suspect word, contagion, would have to be used to describe this fact.[17] With yellow fever, one seemed never able to escape qualifications.

But Dutroulau shared Mélier's outlook. Theory was desirable, but action was essential. A sanitary program had to be built and, if necessary, built upon incomplete information and uncertain theoretical principles. Referring to the confusions of etiology, Dutroulau wrote that "these many qualifications will not please those persons who like to resolve all the problems of epidemiology with mathematical nicety; to me, however, they appear to stem from the very nature of the subject itself. They are sufficient, too, to put before us the obligation of imposing sanitary measures against the chance of importing the disease aboard an infected ship."[18]

In the end, Fonssagrives, Dutroulau, and Mélier had no coherent solution to the etiological problem. Moreover, they had to renounce the aspiration of founding hygienic science upon a solution to that problem. This might be regarded as a useful if unwanted retreat before the etiological issue, a sensible course perhaps for men of active persuasion. Some physicians, however, simply refused to renounce the need to solve the riddle of the cause of yellow fever; to them, the etiological issue was the central issue, from which, once a clear answer had been established, all else would follow. One such figure was Wilhelm Griesinger. Griesinger stated his convictions in almost peremptory manner. "It is apparent at first glance," he announced, "that the classification of infectious diseases is [to be] made according to *etiological principles*. Given the current status of our science, we can conceive how relapsing fever, typhoid fever, Asiatic cholera, yellow fever and the plague are each caused by the host organism taking up a specific poisonous (infective) substance."[19]

In addition to his extensive medical practice in Germany, Griesinger had had firsthand experience with a broad range of exotic diseases. Between 1850 and 1852 he had directed the medical services of the Egyptian government. In that country, supported by his associate and successor, Theodor Bilharz, he had conducted extensive research on the common dis-

17. A. F. Dutroulau, *Traité des maladies des Européens dans les pays chauds (régions tropiques). Climatologie et maladies communes, maladies endémiques* (Paris: J. B. Baillière, 1868), pp. 427–435.

18. Ibid., p. 445.

19. Wilhelm Griesinger, *Infectionskrankheiten, Malariakrankheiten, gelbes Fieber, Typhus, Pest, Cholera* [Rudolf Virchow, ed., *Handbuch der speciellen Pathologie und Therapie*, Bd. II, 2te Abteilung], 2d ed. (Erlangen: F. Enke, 1864), p. 1.

eases of the Nile Valley. (Griesinger admitted, however, to never having seen a case of yellow fever.)[20] Some years after his return from Egypt, and just before he turned to neuropathology and psychiatry, specialties to which he made fundamental contributions, he published his *Infectionskrankheiten*. This remarkable work constituted a massive section of Rudolf Virchow's *Handbuch der speciellen Pathologie und Therapie* and provided a comprehensive, lucid, and critical view of its varied subject matter, an influential *summa* of the subject issued just as the germ theory of disease was beginning to take form.

Griesinger believed that specificity of cause was an idea supported by a host of clinical, pathological, and epidemiological observations; it was the guiding theme of the *Infectionskrankheiten*. "It is the etiological event, . . . the specific intoxication, that renders each infectious disease a distinct entity and separates it from other such entities."[21] Griesinger expected that this notion of specific intoxication provided the means to reduce, even remove, the clash of doctrine that had so long divided contagionist and noncontagionist.

> What is most telling is the process of poisonous infection by means of specific substances. This process calls forth the contagious development of such diseases as the typhus-typhoid fevers, cholera or the plague. In the case of plague we have even succeeded in transferring the poison by means of inoculation. We must assume, furthermore, from the complete similarity of effects between the disease process in the contagious and in the so-called spontaneous or miasmatic diseases that the cause of the latter is of the same kind as the cause of the former; in both cases, we have to postulate an infection by a poison. Whether this cause springs directly from the sick individual (contagion) or whether it arises and then spreads independently of the presence of sick parties, thus arising in the air or soil, in short, in external nature (miasma), it must be of one and the same specific nature because it produces one and the same specific disease.[22]

Pasteur's work appeared to confirm this interpretation. Griesinger appreciated immediately the extraordinary importance of the French chemist's discovery of a series of different fermentations, each mediated by a specific microbe. For Griesinger, this idea — in the language of the chemical etiology of the time, a theory of "zymosis" — replaced previous specu-

20. Ibid., p. 73. On Griesinger in Egypt, see Alexander Mette, *Wilhelm Griesinger. Der Begründer der wissenschaftlichen Pyschiatrie in Deutschland* (Leipzig: B. G. Teubner, 1976), pp. 42–46.

21. Griesinger, *Infectionskrankheiten*, p. 5.

22. Ibid., p. 2. Although making careful distinctions among its members, Griesinger favored the global expression "typhoide Krankheiten" or family of "typhoidal" fevers.

lative ideas regarding etiology. Better yet, "the theory of zymosis has become precisely the same as the [old] theories of miasma and contagion animatum."[23] Nonetheless, he had to admit that all of these novelties, however conducive to furthering the creation of a secure scientific understanding of the cause of infectious diseases, did not wholly eliminate the need to use the traditional adjectives "contagious" and "miasmatic." These, however, did not designate distinct groupings of diseases: they were terms to be used in conjunction with other characteristic features of any given disease.

Griesinger had opened the *Infectionskrankheiten* with brief but powerful general remarks regarding etiology and the promising new era in its study that had just begun. But when he turned to analysis of the nature and behavior of individual communicable diseases, he found that seemingly self-evident theoretical propositions were not easily applied to the messy world of experience. Yellow fever, in particular, confounded his happy expectations. Not knowing the disease firsthand, Griesinger was compelled to follow a literary and comparative approach, testing yellow fever in the light of the epidemic character of more familiar communicable diseases.

It was obvious, he announced, that yellow fever was a miasmatic disease. The association with tropical ports, with ships at sea that had carried no sick when leaving port, and with the vagaries of latitude and seasons, indicated the primacy of local conditions.[24] Nonetheless, while it

23. Ibid., p. 3. Others, however, felt the matter to be anything but resolved. Fernand Monoyer, in a superb review of the subject, concluded: "We need not repeat all of the arguments that have been offered in favor of one or another viewpoint. Facts alone can provide the basis of our theories and, unfortunately for us, experience is silent on this matter. The truth is, we know of all these pathological ferments, viruses, miasmata and the like only because of the morbid symptoms they provoke in the animal economy. We know nothing of the substances on which they act and nothing of how they transform these substances. Here, then, is a cause of profound obscurity and uncertainty, a cause, we must admit, inherent in the imperfect state of our science and in the real difficulties of that science." *Des fermentations. Thèse présentée à la Faculté de médecine de Strasbourg*, 2e série, No. 524 (Strasburg: G. Silbermann, 1862), pp. 148–149. On the zymotic theory, see John Burdon-Sanderson, "On the Intimate Pathology of Contagion," i.e., Appendix No. 11, pp. 229–256, in *Parliamentary Papers* 38 (1870) [Reports from Commissioners. 27. Convict Prisons. Convict Prisons (Ireland). Public Health; i.e., Twelfth Report of the Medical Officer of the Privy Council, with Appendices]; also J. M. Eyler, *Victorian Social Medicine. The Ideas and Methods of William Farr* (Baltimore: Johns Hopkins University Press, 1979), pp. 97–122; Margaret Pelling, *Cholera, Fever and English Medicine, 1825–1865* (Oxford: Oxford University Press, 1978), pp. 100–108, 136–145. The zymotic theory and the new theory of disease germs could approach very near to one another: see E. Rochefort, "Jaune (Fièvre)," *Dictionnaire encyclopédique des sciences médicales*, 100 vols. (Paris: Victor Masson, P. Asselin, 1869–1889), 52:677–678.

24. Griesinger, *Infectionskrankheiten*, p. 80. Griesinger entertained no doubt that the

was true that it had been repeatedly demonstrated that the cause of the disease was the "general genius epidemicus" associated with a particular port or ship or other location, there was also much evidence indicating that the "cause of yellow fever can proceed from a sick individual and can be transmitted by sick individuals."[25] This meant that yellow fever was, to some unspecified degree, contagious as well as noncontagious. Like Fonssagrives and Dutroulau, Griesinger was forced to admit that yellow fever might be transmitted in two ways, even if one (infection via miasma) seemed the typical course and the other (contagion) a rare yet real exception. The possible existence of specific infective agents, microscopic chemical or perhaps living agents, did not allow Griesinger, any more than it did the French investigators, to escape the usual categorization of yellow fever: it was both predominantly noncontagious and somewhat contagious.

These conclusions were in seeming accord with available evidence. Depending upon the case or epidemic examined, evidence was found that tied the outbreak to sharply changed local conditions or to the arrival of a foreign influence, such as a ship from a tropical port. At the same time, it had been demonstrated a thousand times over that personal contact alone did not spread the disease. But other investigators cited instances that supported the latter and denied the former. Chervin had made these questions central to all discussion of yellow fever. He had, in fact, laid down a challenge to his opponents and successors, a challenge, he was confident, that could not be met.[26]

The best opportunity to analyze the cause or causes of individual cases of yellow fever under seemingly controlled conditions appeared to be to observe the circumstances under which susceptible persons, entering an infected area for the first time, contracted the disease. Such cases abounded, particularly in the Antilles where a succession of unacclimatized European arrivals provided the principal fodder for the disease. Chervin asked, How had these individuals made contact with yellow fever? There could have been person-to-person contact and thence direct transmission. But in countless instances person-to-person contact produced no new cases. Moreover, and this was Chervin's challenge, simply by entering the dangerous region these susceptibles were also exposed to an infected atmosphere. At-

---

miasma in question was a "Miasma Animatum," a living agent that arose from or at least was communicated by favorable conditions in the nonliving environment and might also arise from or be communicated by a sick individual. "Miasma Animatum" is excellent witness to both the easy confusion of etiological categories and the infiltration during the 1850s and 1860s of an overtly biological view of disease causation.

25. Ibid., p. 81.

26. Mélier ("Relation de la fièvre jaune survenue à Saint-Nazaire," p. 88) reports this challenge; I have been unable to locate its statement in Chervin's writings.

mospheric contact was inevitable, personal contact at most occasional. He therefore demanded that until one can demonstrate that transmission has occurred well outside such an infected region and by the intermediary of a previously infected individual located in this remote region (i.e., by a person who passes the infection on to another individual who has had no contact whatsoever with that region) there can be no solid grounds for claiming person-to-person transmission. The ports of the Antilles, like ships at sea, would not satisfy this demand. The atmosphere of these ports and their surrounding regions, and all the more so that of a ship sailing from these regions, was by definition infected. No truly isolated case of yellow fever uniquely connected by human contact with other cases of the disease could be found under such circumstances.

In a locality where the disease was not endemic and where the outbreak was limited in scale and its (apparently) relevant parameters were thoroughly understood, such person-to-person transmission might be recognized. Perhaps it could even be proved. Mélier was on the lookout for such an instance; the death of Alphonse Chaillon offered an excellent opportunity to weigh the matter. Indeed, Mélier admitted, this was "the difficult point, I am tempted to say the delicate point, in [my] considerations, [for here one arrives] at the question of the *transmission of the disease from person to person*."[27] But the case of Chaillon seemed unequivocal and Chervin's challenge could be successfully answered.

The circumstances of Chaillon's death had been such, Mélier urged, that an "experimenter who [might] have attempted to conduct such a test would not have carried it out in any way differently" than what actually took place at Saint-Nazaire and Montoir.[28] This was high praise, the experimental ideal by 1860 and not least in France having become an emblem of sound science and an assurance of right reasoning. It meant, too, that the lamented Alphonse Chaillon had become a hard scientific fact, although as Mélier acknowledged, Chaillon constituted the only such known fact.

Unfortunately, this fact was not enough. Chaillon's case only fortified the claim that yellow fever was *also* a contagious disease. Despite the importance of this fact and despite the disproportionate emphasis given it by its discoverer, another and more general fact remained unshaken: yellow fever was predominantly a noncontagious disease. Mélier thus had to read a caution even to himself:

> One must be very careful not to exaggerate the consequences. If it follows, and I believe it does, that the great law that Chervin wished to promul-

27. Ibid., p. 87.
28. Ibid., p. 88.

gate [that is, noncontagionism] is not as true in an absolute sense as he so profoundly thought it to be, it remains a fact that his law holds true in a majority of cases. The events at Saint-Nazaire show that, as before, the transmission [of yellow fever] from person to person must be considered an exceptional event in our climate. Yet it is an exception it would be rash for us, especially those of us concerned with [sanitary] administration, not to take into most serious consideration.[29]

Chervin's challenge had been met, but the accomplishment afforded little satisfaction. Epidemiology had moved no closer to knowledge of the cause of yellow fever. The dual character of the disease asserted itself once again. The definition of sanitary measures, although rendered more precise, had to be such that a nation was protected simultaneously on two fronts: disinfection would be directed to a suspected ship and, more briefly, its cargo; while isolation and observation were to be the lot of passengers and crew. The character of these measures had been established by epidemiological analysis, not by a solution to the etiological enigma.

Missing Victims

Contagionists faced a serious problem, that of missing victims. Without the notion of contact-communication, the category "contagion" had no meaning. Thus, observed the distinguished French clinician Jean Baptiste Bouillaud, it is evident "that the only characteristic that distinguishes contagion from infection . . . is that the former assumes that the disease is transmitted from the sick individual to a healthy individual, whereas the latter refers to the action exerted by infected places upon a more or less sizable number of healthy persons."[30]

The contagionists' dilemma was obvious. What, for example, becomes of a disease which, by definition transmitted from person to person, chances not to meet a receptive new host? Will that disease simply disappear? Must it then arise *de novo*, exhibiting again all of its earlier clinical and pathological characteristics? Could the disease persist but do so without making itself evident in a new victim? The same questions must be answered if one replaces the term *disease* with *causal agent* or *principle of disease*.

Contagious diseases thus seemed to require a continuity of living hosts, although in instance after instance this continuity could not be demonstrated. The affair at Saint-Nazaire offered a striking example of events that could not be satisfactorily embraced by current medical understand-

29. Ibid., p. 90.
30. J. B. Bouillaud, "Contagion," in *Dictionnaire de médecine et de chirurgie pratiques*, 15 vols., ed. Gabriel Andral et al. (Paris: Méquiquon-Marvis, 1829–1836), 3:429.

ing. Upon arrival, the *Anne-Marie* carried a few convalescents but no sick crewmen. Since all crew members of the *Anne-Marie* had not contracted the disease and since these men had lived in close proximity to one another for over six weeks, it was most unlikely that yellow fever was transmitted person-to-person. Moreover, since the disease did in fact manifest itself anew at Saint-Nazaire, and since available evidence demanded that its cause had been imported, the means of importation, not being a sick individual or individuals, had to be the ship itself (or its cargo). It followed that yellow fever had crossed the Atlantic Ocean and it had done so without the continuous presence of living hosts.

For some two weeks after leaving Havana the *Anne-Marie* carried no hosts at all; her entire crew remained quite healthy. An epidemic then broke out, one affecting many members of the crew. This epidemic, however, came to a close while the ship was still at sea and no new cases appeared during the several days before Saint-Nazaire was reached. After only a few days in port, a new wave of disease began. In this sequence of events, human hosts had appeared three times: in Havana, where the crew of the *Anne-Marie* was exposed to a human population in which yellow fever was rapidly spreading; in midvoyage; and among a new population in a virgin port. Human hosts had twice been absent, and this for no short period of time: early in the voyage and during the period prior to arrival. These epidemiological facts seemed to confirm important etiological points: the continuity of human hosts could be interrupted, yellow fever could reassert its presence, the contagionist hypothesis was without merit.

But yellow fever in Saint-Nazaire, and presumably also in Gibraltar, Lisbon, Barcelona, Swansea, or wherever else one cared to look, was the same disease "here" as it was "there." Crucial to the entire analysis was the clinical unity, thus identity of the disease wherever found. As Griesinger had said, one and the same specific disease demands a cause of the same specific nature. Surely there had to be some continuity, "something" that moved from an infected to an uninfected land. Importationists identified this "something" as a specific atmosphere or miasma, trapped within a ship but free to emerge when appropriate conditions presented themselves.

The missing victim phenomenon finds its place within the contagionist-noncontagionist conflict. Rigorously pursued, the contagionist position required that the crew of the *Anne-Marie* fall ill with yellow fever. Close living on a small ship meant close contact with the ill. Of course, caprice of contact might have spared some persons. Perhaps, too, some members of the crew had had previous experience with the disease and were therefore immune, although Mélier made no reference to this possibility. However, this surely had not been the case with the ship's second officer, who fell ill and died in Saint-Nazaire many days after the appearance of the last new case at sea.

Trousseau, an astute observer of all communicable disease, assured his students in his lectures that the invisible germ of contagious diseases could not lead an "independent life." This germ, he continued, demands "an organized and living substratum not only for its existence but no less to give evidence of its existence."[31] If yellow fever were a truly contagious disease, its cause would have to pass from person to person, no other hosts being known, and its presence would be obvious from the constant presence of disease in the exposed population (although, perhaps, not among all members of that population).[32] On the importationist hypothesis, those who fell ill in Saint-Nazaire constituted an exposed population, but they could not have received the disease through contact with sick individuals; there were no sick men aboard *Anne-Marie.* And yet a fast-moving epidemic developed and at least one instance of contact-transmission was identified.

The situation seemed ripe for a contingent-contagionist interpretation. One might feel confident about understanding how an infectious disease such as Asiatic cholera or typhoid fever, but not about how contagious diseases such as smallpox and syphilis, might arise under the influence of unsanitary local conditions. But if an outbreak was uncommonly severe, it seemed that the system of transmission could change dramatically. A disease would give increasing evidence of moving directly from person to person. Trousseau stated this interpretation very clearly. Within a large assemblage of men and women gathered in an insalubrious locale the specific morbific poison of typhoid fever could easily be generated.

> This morbid germ, born spontaneously under conditions set by the nonliving world and then elaborated within living organisms, is passed by contagion to other persons who are not exposed to the conditions which first generated the disease. Now acting alone, contagion spreads typhoid fever not only in the land of its birth but in countries hundreds of miles away.[33]

Contingent contagionism seemed especially useful in explaining such far-moving epidemics and reinterpreting more localized epidemics that affected large numbers of persons. This theory was frequently applied to familiar

31. Armand Trousseau, *Clinique médicale de l'Hôtel-Dieu,* 2 vols., ed. A. Vanmotti et al. (Geneva: Alliance culturelle du livre, 1963), 1:371.

32. Mélier explicitly excluded the role of rats in the transmission of yellow fever: "Relation de la fièvre jaune survenue à Saint-Nazaire," pp. 76–77. Fonssagrives (*Traité de l'hygiène navale*) reviews the question.

33. Trousseau, *Clinique médicale de l'Hôtel-Dieu* 1:378. See the summary argument in Pelling, *Cholera, Fever and English Medicine,* pp. 295–310.

epidemic diseases and it was common coin to interpreters of yellow fever as well.

Mélier possessed but a single instance of contagion, albeit a seemingly indubitable one, and he had neither need nor inclination to adopt a contingent-contagionist interpretation of yellow fever. At most, he granted that the facts at Saint-Nazaire "seemed to show . . . that yellow fever, while incontestably an imported disease, might to a certain degree also be transmissible" by contagion.[34] The heart of the contingent-contagionist solution—that is, given time, numerous victims, and an intense infection, a disease produced by a noncontagious agent could give rise to a specific contagious agent—found no place in his discussion. He simply accepted the dual causal character of yellow fever and made no attempt to explain it. He was not bound by the contagionist's need for a continuity of living hosts and thus had no particular problem with missing victims of the disease.

Obviously, nothing at Saint-Nazaire advanced understanding of the nature of the causal agent of yellow fever. Nor did subsequent microscopical investigation offer satisfaction. Mélier could offer, however, conclusions of practical importance. Yellow fever is an importable disease; it exhibits both noncontagious and contagious qualities; its spread can be checked by timely application of appropriate sanitary measures. I have, he stated, "often read the reports of various epidemics." I have reread them all "in response to the events at Saint-Nazaire. I must say that the more I study these reports, the more I am struck by the evidence supporting the following propositions: . . . [with regard to yellow fever, we must accept] *origin by importation,* subsequent *spread and propagation,* to which sick individuals make a contribution and the *necessity of sanitary measures.* Around precisely these three propositions argument has long raged and Chervin devoted both his life and his fortune to attacking them: he rejected them all."[35]

But Chervin, now hapless in memory, was proved wrong. Local conditions had no role in the development of a yellow-fever epidemic unless the specific miasmatic agent of that disease had been introduced into the locality in question. Despite the fact that the nature of the infecting agent remained unknown, there was now proof that it moved with ships. Chervin had feared no arriving ship, however dangerous its port of origin or sickly its crew. Mélier had learned to fear only certain ships, and as a consequence formulated measures that would reduce and perhaps eliminate the risk by ensuring that yellow fever, should it reach the coastal waters of France, could not come ashore.

34. Mélier, "Relation de la fièvre jaune survenue à Saint-Nazaire," p. 115.
35. Ibid., p. 96.

Such was the lesson of Saint-Nazaire and the formal end to the French experiment with drastically reduced control over maritime access to her Atlantic ports. A few years later, and not at all far away, equally careful scientific inquiry generated very similar epidemiological conclusions and etiological confusions. There was little change, however, in public sanitary action. Still, if yellow fever at Swansea was obviously the same disease, it had entered a very different nation.

6

Swansea, 1865

EPIDEMIC YELLOW FEVER reached Swansea in the late summer of 1865. It did not linger long, but there was sufficient time for two dozen local residents to fall ill with the disease and for two-thirds of these victims to die. Never before had Britain suffered such an epidemic, and she would not be bothered again. While the experience caused only momentary public alarm, it provoked an epidemiological inquiry of major historical interest.

The first indication of trouble was the appearance of James Saunders, a seaman aboard the sailing ship *Hecla*. Seriously ill upon arrival in Swansea, Saunders was taken ashore on the morning of 9 September. He died at noon on the same day. William Clouston, master of the *Hecla*, had declared to port authorities that Saunders suffered from dropsy. Swansea medical opinion, however, quickly rejected that self-serving conclusion; the reported cause of death was stated to be "fever, probably yellow fever." Other observers shared this conclusion and recognized the seriousness of the situation. John Simon in London, for example, noted that the events at Swansea constituted "an entirely new phenomenon," one that required immediate and exacting inquiry.[1] Simon was Medical Officer of the Privy Council, a position of modest influence but great visibility, and it was his responsibility to assure that a proper investigation was carried out. He assigned this task to George Buchanan, who was then at the outset of what was to become a distinguished career in the emerging public-medical services of Great Britain.

Buchanan traveled to Swansea and there explored the varied and contradictory aspects of the epidemic. His inquiry was thorough but his report brief. Buchanan's conclusions regarding the origin and movement of the epidemic in Swansea were virtually identical to those reached by Fran-

1. John Simon, "III. Foreign Epidemics of the Year and the General Question of Contagion in its Bearings on the Public Health. 3. Yellow Fever at Swansea," *Parliamentary Papers* 33 (1866) [Reports from Commissioners. 17. Pollution of Rivers. Public Health; i.e., Eighth Report of the Medical Officer of the Privy Council, with Appendices, 1865], p. 30. For an account of the Swansea yellow-fever epidemic and a detailed modern assessment of factors bearing on the movement of the disease, see C. E. Gordon Smith and M. E. Gibson, "Yellow Fever in South Wales, 1865," *Medical History* 30 (1986): 322–340.

çois Mélier regarding yellow fever in Saint-Nazaire. Nonetheless, although Buchanan and Simon were well acquainted and largely in agreement with the Frenchman's assessment of events in Brittany, British and French views differed significantly on the matter of the measures to be used to reduce the threat of yellow fever.

Buchanan worked within a British framework of radically reduced provisions for quarantine. Such action as might be taken was the responsibility of local officials, not of the central government, and these local officials were limited by law as to what they might do. Recent national experience was hardly encouraging. While plague remained absent and posed no test to the faltering quarantine machinery, by 1865 Asiatic cholera had entered Britain three times despite valiant efforts to close all ports to the visitor. Quarantine in Britain was not a matter of high regard, suffering repeated criticism in principle and widespread neglect in practice. Parliament was pleased with these developments, the Commons resolving that "this House approves of the various relaxations of the [quarantine] laws and regulations which have from time to time been introduced, and desires that such further relaxations may be urged upon the attention of foreign Governments and adopted at home, as may be found compatible with a due regard to the public health and the commercial interests of the community."[2] Other public agencies thought similarly. British coastal defense continued to be sanitary defense — deploying disinfection as its primary weapon — and was limited in its reach by legislative restraints upon the competence of central administrative authority; officers of the French government enjoyed wider powers and were less bemused by a strictly sanitary view of communicable disease.

George Buchanan (1831–1895) was born and trained in London.[3] He served as resident and consulting physician to the London Fever Hospital and then, receiving an appointment as Medical Officer of Health to the St. Giles district of the metropolis, gradually began to emphasize public-health activity. During the 1860s he worked on an occasional basis for the medical department of the Privy Council, conducting a number of influential specialized investigations, of which that at Swansea was one; in 1869 he became a permanent inspector. He continued this connection when the Privy Council's medical responsibilities were taken over by the

2. "Report on Quarantine by the Committee of the National Association for the Promotion of Social Science, with Appendix," in *Parliamentary Papers* 58 (1861) [Accounts and Papers. 25. Shipping and Trade. No. 544. Papers relating to Quarantine communicated to the Board of Trade on the 30th Day of July 1861], p. 47.
3. R. T. T. [R. T. Thorne], [George Buchanan], *Proceedings of the Royal Society* 59 (1895–1896): xli–xliii; Anon., "Sir George Buchanan, M.D., L.L.D., F.R.S.," *Transactions of the Epidemiological Society*, n.s., 14 (1894–1895): 113–117.

new Local Government Board (1871), becoming principal Medical Officer of the board in 1879 and serving in that position until his retirement in 1892.

This broad medical experience had made Buchanan familiar with the common communicable diseases of the British Isles. He knew Asiatic cholera, too, from the epidemic of 1854–1855, but it was for him an entirely new experience to examine cases of yellow fever and this in so unlikely a setting as Wales. Novelty, nonetheless, evoked no serious doubts. All evidence indicated that the Swansea affliction was "no ordinary English fever," and it was also not relapsing fever, which had been previously met in Swansea but did not represent the danger inherent in the new fever. In Buchanan's view, the only possible conclusion was that here in the Welsh port there was "bonâ fide the West Indian yellow fever itself."[4] Scarlatina, diphtheria, and smallpox were common enough in Swansea, but 1865 was not a year of serious activity for these well-characterized diseases. Malarial fevers were very rare in the locality.

The new disease exhibited distinguishing diagnostic features. Buchanan cited especially the sudden onset, severe headache and lower back pain, continued high fever, black vomit and jaundice, suppression of urine, and mental alertness until the end. The end came quickly, often on the third day of illness. As a consequence of these observations, it was confidently concluded that Swansea had been struck by a specific and novel disease, a disease truly without local origins. Local physicians immediately called it yellow fever, and Buchanan and Simon soon afterwards did the same.[5] Their conclusion was but a prelude to another, namely, this was an imported disease. Once again, attention was directed to determining just

4. "Report by Dr. George Buchanan on the Outbreak of Yellow Fever at Swansea," *Parliamentary Papers* 33 (1866) [note 1, above], p. 450.

5. Ibid., pp. 442–443. But local opinion was not unanimous and certain singularities were noted. Thus, a Dr. Paddon of Swansea (ibid., p. 443n.) observed that after arrival of an unhealthy ship from Havana local gastric fevers tended to become more intense and delirium more severe; Paddon's claim may be only a product of his imagination or, a reasonable likelihood, he may have observed subacute cases of yellow fever (which possibility raises the question, were there on these occasions no acute cases of the disease?). It is possible that another Swansea physician (Dr. Griffith[s]), who attended several of the earliest victims and soon thereafter fell seriously ill, had contracted yellow fever; however, neither Buchanan nor, apparently, the victim himself regarded the sickness as being yellow fever (ibid., p. 466). The specificity of yellow fever and thus the fact of importation were denied by J. R. Cormack, "What Is the Nature of the 'Yellow' Fever Now at Swansea?," *British Medical Journal* 2 (1865): 381–382, 430–432, 512–513, and vigorously reasserted by George Padley, "The Yellow Fever in Swansea," ibid., pp. 459–460. A. P. Wilks, "The Cases of Yellow Fever at Swansea," *Lancet* 2 (1865): 495–496, emphasized the distinctiveness of the disease. Padley and Wilks were Swansea practitioners, the former Senior Physician to the Swansea Infirmary, and the latter attended one of the first victims until his death; Cormack was a London practitioner. It may

how such an exotic disease had gained access to a remote northern port. Buchanan, like Mélier four years earlier, attended principally to the epidemiology of the disease. Nonetheless, he — and especially Simon, who observed and commented at length on the inquiry — found it difficult, in fact, impossible, not to confound epidemiological conclusions and etiological questions. Once again, uncertainty ensued.

The Case of the *Hecla*

Swansea in 1865 was a major British industrial city.[6] Lying on the edge of the South Wales coal field, she had been a leading metallurgical center since the late seventeenth century. The city's specialty was the smelting of nonferrous metals, especially copper. It was economically more attractive to bring copper ore to Swansea, where coal for smelting was abundant and cheap, than to attempt to reduce the ore near the mines themselves. As a result, by the mid-nineteenth century Swansea provided 90 percent of Britain's copper and accounted for over 50 percent of world production of the metal.

Originally ore from nearby mines, principally in Cornwall, was used. But by 1840 British ore was rapidly becoming noncompetitive as new and far richer deposits were discovered and gradually brought into production. Chilean, Australian, and North American mines soon shifted the character of the copper trade and new maritime connections were established with those regions. This trade followed northern or far southern routes and in the New World centered on ports generally well removed from the endemic yellow-fever zone. Somewhat earlier, however, copper ore had begun to be imported through Swansea from Cuba. The leading British importer, the Cobre Mining Association, exploited property in the southeastern corner of the island, and its ships sailed to Swansea from the port of Santiago de Cuba. At latitude 20°00′N., the Cuban port was very much within the yellow-fever zone.

The *Hecla* was a small wooden sailing ship belonging to the Cobre Association. Carrying a clean bill of health, she sailed from Santiago de Cuba on 26 July 1865 and passed, with her cargo of copper ore, directly

---

be noted that no postmortems of the Swansea dead were conducted. It was Paddon who pressed London authorities to initiate an inquiry into the epidemic: Buchanan, "Report on Yellow Fever at Swansea," p. 447.

6. See R. O. Roberts, "The Development and Decline of the Non-Ferrous Metal Smelting Industries in South Wales," in *Industrial South Wales, 1750–1914. Essays in Welsh Economic History*, ed. W. E. Minchinton (London: Frank Cass, 1969), pp. 121–160; W. G. V. Balchin, ed., *Swansea and Its Region* (Swansea: University College of Swansea for the British Association for the Advancement of Science, 1971).

to Swansea.[7] She reached the Bristol Channel on the evening of 8 September and there the channel pilots and then the port pilots came aboard. The master of the *Hecla*, Clouston, told the Swansea pilot that he had lost three men at sea from sickness and that another seaman, Saunders, was seriously ill. Clouston requested supplementary crew members; five new men came aboard. In all of this, he made no reference to yellow fever. The Swansea pilot, suspecting nothing, brought the *Hecla* into the North Dock, located in the heart of the city, arriving there at nine o'clock on the morning of 9 September.

Once again, a Cuban ship brought both wealth and trouble to a European port. Within an hour the crew and the two passengers had disembarked and moved into the town, taking their personal goods with them. Three crew members "were landed sick": two, it was said, were "recovering from 'fever'" and the third, again Saunders, was said to have dropsy.[8] The ship's hatches were opened and unloading of the cargo was begun within a few hours of arrival; everything concerning the ship appeared to be normal.

Nonetheless, the *Hecla* aroused the suspicion of some observers whose anxieties gained sound foundation when Saunders died a few hours after landing. Warned by the port's sanitary inspector of the unhealthy condition aboard the *Hecla*, the mayor of Swansea and a local physician visited Saunders in the filthy hovel in Welcome Court to which he had been removed (see map location B). Two physicians had visited him somewhat earlier. One of these men had seen yellow-fever cases abroad and declared Saunders to be ill with this disease. Saunders' second pair of visitors had scarcely left when a message was sent them saying that the victim had died. The cause of death was certified to be "fever, probably yellow fever."[9] Upon subsequent inquiry, the master of the *Hecla* conceded that the deaths at sea aboard his ship were probably also due to yellow fever.

There was nothing unusual in these several events. Many a ship's master had failed to declare his suspicions of the character of the disease that ravaged his vessel during the crossing from America. The master of the *Dygden* had certainly not called attention to the potentially serious unhealthy condition of his ship upon arrival in Gibraltar, and Captain Voisin of the *Anne-Marie* reported to authorities in Saint-Nazaire only that a colic had attacked his men. Furthermore, yellow fever had visited Swansea in previous years. In 1843, 1851, and 1864 (and perhaps on other occa-

7. The following account of events aboard the *Hecla* is taken from Buchanan, "Report on Yellow Fever at Swansea," pp. 444–448.

8. Ibid., p. 445.

9. Ibid. This determination was made by Paddon, who was engaged with caring for victims of the epidemic from the outset.

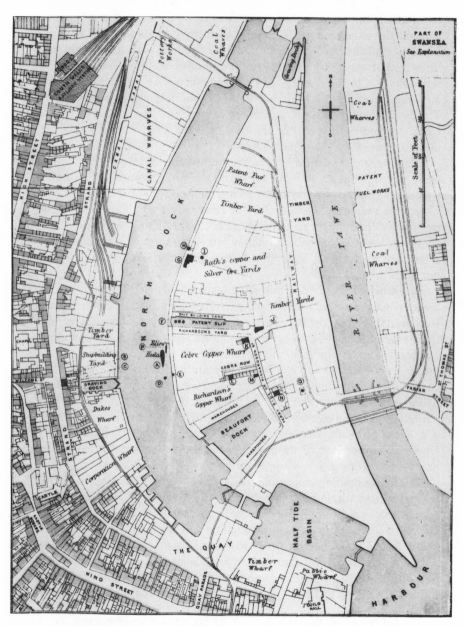

Map of the North Dock and Island, Swansea, 1865. Location A shows the position of the *Hecla* on 9 September; location P shows the position of the *Eleanor* while taking on cargo. Locations B–O indicate residences or places of employment of victims of yellow fever. (*Parliamentary Papers* 33 [1866] (Reports from Commissioners. 17. Pollution of Rivers. Public Health), following p. 468.)

sions) the Saunders phenomenon had occurred, that is, an ailing crewman/passenger came ashore, there to die of his complaint (yellow fever). Death at sea, too, was not uncommon aboard Swansea ships trading with Cuba; in 1865, two ships besides the *Hecla* lost members of their crews, presumably to yellow fever.

The principal contrast between the events occasioned by yellow fever at Swansea and at Saint-Nazaire is seen in the actions taken by port authorities hoping to check the spread of the disease. Whatever their shortcomings, French sanitary regulations permitted early and extensive interference in the affairs of shipping. British administrative powers regarding private property were more limited. With regard to Saunders' body, his final resting place, and the persons and effects of other crewmen and passengers, immediate and vigorous action was possible. The dead man was quickly buried; the clothing and the bodies of the living were disinfected with chlorine fumes; and rooms were cleaned, disinfected, and whitewashed.

Local authorities, naturally enough, were "further desirous of dealing with the *Hecla* herself, on the supposition that she might be a source of infection." This posed a more serious challenge. The *Hecla* was private property and the Swansea agent for the Cobre Association strongly opposed any interference with the routine of unloading the cargo and preparing the ship for return to Cuba. He cited the experience of thirty years, during which regular communication with Santiago de Cuba had been maintained and no ill effects had befallen the inhabitants of Swansea. Local magistrates, customs authorities, and the Swansea board of health examined the matter and, while agreeing that the *Hecla* should never have entered the port, "found themselves powerless to insist on her removal."[10] British law permitted no direct assault on the perceived source of the threat.

But indirect action was possible and this was undertaken on command of the municipal authorities. The town police were ordered to remove all persons from the ship and prevent others from boarding her. This, obviously, halted unloading of the *Hecla*'s cargo and established, it appears, a more compliant attitude on the part of the Cobre agent. Disinfection of the ship could now begin and soon thereafter unloading started anew.

During this first or preepidemic period in Swansea (9–15 September) several confused inquiries were conducted into the condition of the *Hecla* upon her arrival, the events surrounding the death of Saunders, and the risk posed to the people of Swansea. These inquiries elicited from Clouston the true state of affairs aboard his unfortunate vessel. They also led the local collector of customs to place the *Hecla* in quarantine.

10. Ibid., p. 446.

What did, or could, this mean? As Buchanan discovered a few weeks later, it did not mean much. The quarantine questions were put to Clouston on the ninth — after the ship's arrival in the North Dock — but, as noted above, he did not at that time report the occurrence of serious disease aboard his ship or in her port of departure. The questions themselves were designed to elicit from the master of a suspect ship a verbal report on the general medical experience of his vessel; they were not backed by interrogation of others or direct inspection of the ship.[11] A ship's master could easily dissimulate and Clouston did so. He had erred, too, in failing to fly the yellow warning flag of quarantine upon entering the port. Furthermore, by the time that suspicions had been thoroughly aroused by Saunders' death, crew members and passengers had disembarked and dispersed. Quarantine, if such were to be contemplated, would have had to proceed without the parties most concerned. Clouston was not alone in sin. The Swansea customs officers, the only relevant local representatives of the central government, had not looked closely; even when trouble quite literally presented itself in the form of the dying Saunders, they still did not initiate protective measures. This was done only by the mayor of Swansea, who attempted to halt all communication with the ship.[12]

The physician who certified Saunders' death from yellow fever demanded a more thorough investigation. His telegram of 9 September to the Board of Trade in London, under whose authority the customs service operated, evoked no response; but a letter sent to the same body two days later brought an inspector from Newport (Mr. Cullum) to look into the entire affair. He arrived on the fifteenth and was obviously a more determined inquirer, carefully reexamining all available evidence and insisting on extracting the truth from Clouston.

11. Simon stated clearly the dubious purpose of these "questions": "It may be proper to mention that the ceremonies to which, under the name of quarantine, certain trans-Atlantic ships are subjected, on their arrival in this country, have not, properly speaking, any medical significance in relation to this country, but are part of an international obligation contracted for commercial reasons" ("Yellow Fever at Swansea," p. 42n.). Simon's comment refers to the following practice: ". . . a great reduction would have been made in the quarantines usually imposed for the plague, had it not been for the vigilant jealousy of the consuls of different nations resident in this country, who immediately reported any alteration in our quarantine practice to their respective Governments, which eagerly seized every opportunity as an excuse for putting all arrivals from this country in quarantine. Of recent years it has been almost exclusively on account of yellow fever, when the disease has actually existed in vessels during the voyage, that quarantine has been exercised; and this has been chiefly at Southampton, in the case of the West India mail steamers," "Report on Quarantine by the Committee of the National Association for the Promotion of Social Science, *Parliamentary Papers* 58 (1861), p. 17. The French government did precisely this in 1865, refusing entry into France of ships from Swansea and Llanelli: Cormack, "What Is the Nature of the 'Yellow' Fever Now at Swansea?," p. 432.

12. Buchanan, "Report on Yellow Fever at Swansea," p. 447.

Cullum submitted his report to the London customs authorities, who then resolved the matter in characteristically bureaucratic manner. They observed:

> There has been great irregularity and neglect of the usual precautions on the part of all persons on board and . . . the master, the Swansea pilot as well as the Bristol [Channel] pilot, and the crew who landed from the vessel have in strictness rendered themselves liable to prosecution under the quarantine laws. They would, however, appear to have acted in ignorance and not from any willful intention of violating the law.[13]

The Board of Customs and then the Privy Council, to which Cullum's report was referred, saw reason to assume culpability on the part of many but chose only to issue a general warning and to prosecute no one.

This was surely a singular conclusion. Buchanan announced in undisguised language what Cullum had established earlier, that the master of the *Hecla* had lied to the first customs officer at Swansea during the latter's inquiry of 9 September. Clouston knew well, and so stated to the second investigator (Cullum), that "sickness," its nature unspecified, had been present aboard the *Hecla* while in Cuba. Moreover, in the record of "Receipts of Wages and Effects," a document which each ship's master was required to keep for seamen who died while in service, Clouston listed the cause of the deaths at sea as "yellow fever."[14]

Two men from the *Hecla* had taken sick while in Cuba and had died there. Three more crewmen died during the crossing, and Saunders died immediately upon reaching Swansea. Since two of the men dead at sea were reported to have been sick for sixteen days and forty-two days, and Saunders' own illness was stated to have lasted fourteen days, it is possible, if these figures are correct, that diseases other than yellow fever had reigned aboard the *Hecla*.[15] Perhaps this fact, or possibility, absolves Clouston of some blame for his false statements to the first customs officer. Furthermore, a disease so easily confused by medical men experienced with other communicable diseases would not be one that a ship's captain, even a master who regularly traveled the Cuba route, could always or authoritatively identify. Clouston, however, did entertain grave suspicions of the sickness aboard his ship and knew very well that the

13. Ibid.
14. Ibid.
15. Ibid. These figures permit no assured conclusions. Convalescence may be prolonged but "after the 10th day, deaths from uncomplicated yellow fever are very rare": J. A. Kerr, "The Clinical Aspects and Diagnosis of Yellow Fever," in *Yellow Fever*, ed. G. K. Strode (New York: McGraw-Hill, 1951), pp. 416–417. David Richards, whose illness was reported to have lasted forty-seven days, must surely have taken sick in Havana itself, for the crossing lasted but thirty-eight days; his is a most improbable case of yellow fever.

Hecla's entry into Swansea and access to her wharfs would be delayed, perhaps for an extended period, if he gave them voice. He said nothing — and no one imposed a penalty for his deception or for neglect on the part of others.

Obviously, this instance represents a test of the intent of any law or administrative ruling. One's measure is not words but enforcement. Some people, but by no means all, thought British arrangements in these matters a veritable scandal. The naval surgeon Alexander Bryson, one of Britain's foremost students of epidemic diseases and especially of yellow fever, told Parliament that a false statement by a ship's master was a very serious offense and one that was vastly compounded when, as a consequence, epidemic disease spread throughout an innocent community. "As the crime is great," he stated, "the penalty against infraction [should] be severe, equal at least to that of manslaughter. This might deter shipmasters and others from attempting, by false means, to evade quarantine."[16] As usual, the legislature did not heed such words; the law contained no necessary sanctions that might have brought Clouston or others to trial. Rather, it was unusual that they received even an administrative rebuke from the Privy Council.

Yellow Fever in Swansea

What is perhaps most remarkable in all of these proceedings is that there had been as yet no epidemic of yellow fever in Swansea. During this first period, Saunders' death had occasioned only desultory investigation and modest sanitary intervention. His illness had not spread to persons unconnected with the voyage. It had not even led to removal of the offending ship from the harbor. The second period, that is, the epidemic itself, began on 15 September but was recognized only a week later.

The affair opened with a worker from the *Hecla* falling ill on the fifteenth. His symptoms included headache, high fever, delirium, and frequent vomiting. These continued for several days and then recovery began. His convalescence was slow; when seen by Buchanan on 1 October, he was still "much jaundiced." Although he resided far from the port, the victim's connection with the *Hecla* was close and easily established. He had boarded the ill-fated ship on the ninth and went aboard twice during the following week. This case, however, received notice only after the event; the victim, after all, recovered.[17] It took death to arouse serious concern.

On 23 September a Swansea physician reported the death of one of

16. Alexander Bryson, in "Report on Quarantine," *Parliamentary Papers* 58 (1861), p. 36.
17. Buchanan, "Report on Yellow Fever at Swansea," p. 458.

his patients to the local board of health. The cause of death was listed as yellow fever. The report was promptly dispatched to the office of the Registrar General in London, from which the news was immediately transmitted to the Medical Officer of the Privy Council. Simon received the report on the twenty-sixth and his representative, Buchanan, was at work in Swansea on the twenty-seventh. He remained there with the exception of one day until 5 October and stayed in regular contact by post with local physicians and others until 23 October, the date his own report was submitted to Simon. By chance, the last death from yellow fever at Swansea occurred on the day of Buchanan's departure from Wales.

Buchanan acted in Swansea much as Mélier had done in Saint-Nazaire. He inspected the suspect ship, visited victims of the disease and interrogated local physicians and town authorities. His role was both investigative and advisory. With regard to investigation, much could be done; with regard to action, the options were far fewer.

Yellow fever progressed rapidly in Swansea. By the time Buchanan reached the city on the twenty-seventh, ten cases had appeared. The death formally reported on the twenty-third had in fact occurred on the twenty-second and on that same day two additional deaths took place. During the entire epidemic (first case, 15 September; last new case, 4 October; first death, 22 September; last death, 5 October), twenty-nine persons were stricken and sixteen died. (Saunders is excluded from these sums.) Assuming that all victims suffered from yellow fever (Buchanan considered seven cases to be "doubtful"), the case-fatality rate was 55 percent. Excluding the doubtful cases, twenty-two persons fell ill and fifteen died, the case-fatality rate now being 68 percent.[18]

The Swansea report reflected the premise of importation. Buchanan's arguments and supporting evidence for his claim were similar to those put forward a few years earlier by Mélier, although he did not attempt to explore the matter in the same wide-ranging manner followed by the French investigator. Several independent arguments were used to indict the *Hecla*.[19] The likelihood of importation was suggested by the fact that a specific disease had suddenly appeared in Swansea, a disease that could not be identified with any of the common local diseases. Moreover, experienced observers of yellow fever recognized that precisely this disease and no other was present in epidemic form. There was continuity, too, between the ailing town and the infected ship. Fever, no doubt yellow fever, had been aboard the *Hecla:* Saunders was the best witness to this fact, and Clous-

18. All cases and deaths are listed in summary form, ibid., p. 449; each is described in detail in the case reports reproduced by Buchanan, ibid., pp. 458–466. The caution may once again be stated that these figures refer to acute cases only; the possible existence and numbers of subacute cases passed without comment.

19. Ibid., pp. 451–452.

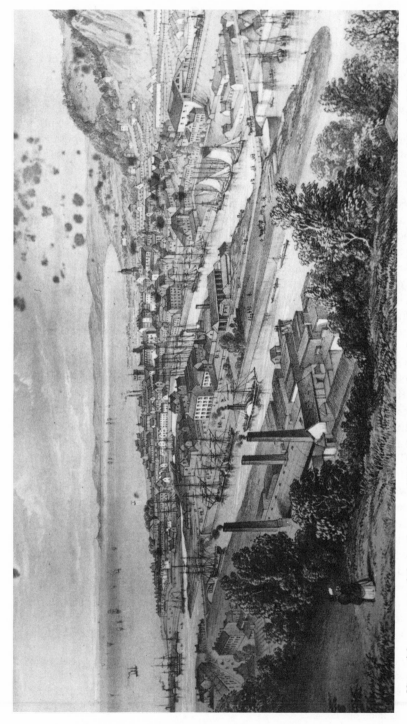

View of Swansea toward the southwest, ca. 1858. In the foreground a smelter and the river Tawe, then the Island and the North Dock; beyond the latter the castle and the old town. The Cobre Mining Association's sheds stand below the cluster of masts in the North Dock; the *Hecla* in 1865 was anchored in the Dock a few yards from these sheds. (Courtesy of the Swansea Museum.)

ton's final admission of serious disease at sea provided further support. Other Swansea ships had experienced yellow fever at sea but, as became clear upon investigation, none except the *Hecla* arrived in a sickly condition during the critical weeks of August and September 1865.

The timing of these events was fully appreciated. On 9 September an infected vessel had entered the port, thus presenting herself to a large susceptible population. Six days later the first local victim was stricken. Furthermore, the *Hecla* was banished from the Beaufort Dock—an enclosed area which opened off the North Dock and within which the *Hecla* was briefly secluded—and tied in isolation to the outer jetty of the harbor on 28 September. The last case of yellow fever occurred on 4 October, just six days after this maneuver. Thus, Buchanan concluded, between 9 September and 4 October, the period of the *Hecla*'s close association with the port of Swansea, numerous "cases of a disease previously unknown at the port [broke] out, with the symptoms and fatality that mark it for yellow fever."[20]

Even more striking was the physical connection that bound victim and ship. Swansea was a middle-sized city (her population in 1861 was 42,581) and was rapidly growing. Local topography was quite varied and the city's economic activity diverse. Yet yellow fever touched only a minute fraction of the population, persons whose residence or work brought them into close daily proximity to the North Dock. Buchanan summarized the evidence as follows:

> Of the 22 cases of fever (excluding doubtful cases of it) that subsequently [broke] out, 11 [occurred] in persons resident on the little island [which separated the North Dock and the river Tawe a few yards to the east; the Cobre wharf stood on the east side of the North Dock: see map]; 5 in persons who, living elsewhere in the town, [had] their daily work on the island, 3 in men occupied about shipping in the North Dock, and only 2 cases [occurred] among the whole population of the large town who had no direct connection with the island. But even these two cases [occurred] in persons living within 150 yards of the ship, across the dock, and living in the next house but one to the cottage where the man died who was taken from the vessel on her arrival.[21]

Two of these several deaths, furthermore, had occurred not in Swansea but in the neighboring port of Llanelli and here, too, lines of connection could be established.

These events are analogous to those manifested earlier in Saint-Nazaire. Unlike the French situation, however, none of the Swansea victims had

20. Ibid., p. 452.
21. Ibid.; population of Swansea, ibid., p. 440.

actually worked aboard the *Hecla* (except, of course, Saunders, whose case, strictly speaking, does not belong to the Swansea epidemic). Nonetheless, many victims in various employments—harbor patrolman, laborer in a shipyard and another in a blacksmith shop, ore carrier, assayer of the ore landed from the *Hecla*—had worked near the ship. Many victims lived on the island and thus close to the North Dock. Several of these persons had visited aboard the *Hecla* and a number of other victims who had not boarded the ship had relatives living at the same address who had done so. Two victims, James Hickey (who recovered) and his wife, Elizabeth (who died), had had, so far as careful inquiry could determine, no connections at all with either the *Hecla* or the island to which she was joined. But their residence on The Strand (see map location C) was directly across the narrow Welcome Court from the house (see map location B) to which Saunders had been taken to die. James and Elizabeth Hickey fell ill on 20 and 22 September, respectively, and the nature of the infectious connection with Saunders, if any, belonged to the mysteries of the disease. Welcome Court and The Strand, however, stood less than five hundred feet from the *Hecla* and thus the Hickeys, Buchanan suggested, might have been the victims of an influence from the ship itself, an influence moving with (or without) human intermediary.

Here again is an instance of numerous epidemiological possibilities with no means by which to choose among them. Buchanan presented meteorological data showing that, from the fourteenth onward, the prevailing winds over the North Dock blew often from the east or northeast. They were therefore ideal for conveying an atmospheric influence from the *Hecla* to Welcome Court, though Buchanan did not address this possibility. He noted, however, that James Hickey did not "see Saunders during life, but that he helped to put the coffin on the cart on the afternoon of the 9th, and he took some whiskey in to the friends of the man, probably before the means of disinfection were used." The movements of Elizabeth Hickey passed unrecorded; she was pregnant when stricken, suffered a miscarriage on the third day of her illness, and died on the fourth. The implication of all this was that a miasmatic influence was active. Other possibilities consistent with nineteenth-century understanding can easily be imagined, and to these the twentieth century adds the role of the mosquito. Buchanan himself speculated that Saunders, who had come "direct from the *Hecla*, . . . might have brought some of her atmosphere with him." The situation is reminiscent of the death of Alphonse Chaillon at Montoir, although in the latter case the distance separating ship and victim was four miles, not five hundred feet.[22]

22. Ibid., pp. 465, 453.

Perhaps the most remarkable event of the Swansea epidemic was the fate of the *Eleanor*. Here was an almost exact repetition of events four years earlier aboard the several vessels which had left Saint-Nazaire for nearby ports. Copper ore received in Swansea was often transshipped, moving, for example, to the combined coal port of Llanelli and metallurgical town of Penclawdd. On 22 September the sloop *Eleanor* arrived at Llanelli, about fifty sea miles west of Swansea, having just discharged her cargo of copper ore at Penclawdd.[23] She had sailed from Swansea on 18–19 September and her crew, all of whom had been with the ship for at least nine months, was in excellent health. Within a week, three members of the crew fell seriously ill and two subsequently died. The history of the first victim, Charles Hayes, is a model of the uncertainty that commonly surrounded death by yellow fever. Healthy on the twenty-second, apparently stricken on the twenty-third, certainly ill on the twenty-fourth, he was dead by early afternoon on the twenty-fifth. No physician visited him and no post-mortem was conducted; it is possible, too, that his complaint was not yellow fever. He died, it appeared, by an act of God. The other victims, one of whom died, were visited by a physician and there seems little doubt that their disease was in fact yellow fever.

But how could this be? How could a healthy crew, moving from one healthy port (as Swansea still appeared to be on 19 September) to another, be so seriously afflicted by an altogether unexpected disease? Only in retrospect did the situation become clear. Buchanan explained these events just as Mélier had explained the movement of yellow fever from Saint-Nazaire to Indret and Lorient. The *Eleanor*, he observed,

> was loaded at Swansea on September 18th. She came to her berth, however, partly inside the *Hecla* (that is, with part of the vessel lying between the *Hecla* and the wharf [see map location P]) on the evening of the 16th, and remained there over the 17th. While taking in her cargo of copper ore, she lay close above the *Hecla*, to the north. This week was just the time the *Hecla* was discharging cargo. No ore from the *Hecla* was taken by the *Eleanor*.[24]

Of these singular facts the laconic Buchanan could only say that they possessed "much interest."[25] Unlike Mélier, he did not insist, nor did Simon do so in his commentary, upon what in such a situation seemed an inevitable conclusion: one ship, here the *Eleanor*, had acquired the principle of yellow fever from and while lying near another ship, the *Hecla*.

Conclusion it was, however, and a very pointed one. Yet Buchanan

23. Ibid., pp. 466–468.
24. Ibid., p. 468.
25. Ibid., p. 452.

possessed, as did virtually every student of yellow fever, other facts that diminished the force of the argument. The case of the *Eleanor*, like that of the *Chastang* (the tug that had moved from Saint-Nazaire to Indret), showed that a disease principle could pass from one population to another and strike down members of both groups; other facts showed that this was not a common occurrence. Thus, not one person among the pilots who had guided the *Hecla* into Swansea, the replacement crew members she had taken aboard, the customs officers who examined her, and the men who had unloaded the ship (so far as the latter could be traced, "most" being known according to Buchanan) contracted yellow fever. Here were at least a dozen local men and probably many more, each of whom may be presumed to have been highly susceptible to the disease, and yet not one new victim appeared. Although it was not stated, the same observation applies to the numerous persons living on the island, working on or near the North Dock, or simply passing through nearby parts of the town — most of whom would also be susceptibles. These were the usual vagaries of yellow fever and they seemed quite beyond explanation.

Despite a resolve not to do so, Mélier and others had followed such suggestive facts into the hopeless tangle of etiological speculation. Buchanan, too, tried to avoid this thicket, again with uncertain success. But for all that, he understood, as Mélier before him had understood, that the facts themselves provided no grounds for exonerating an infected ship, in this case, the *Hecla*. With reference to the perplexing matter of the absence of expected victims, Buchanan acknowledged that "no [causal] explanation can yet be offered," and noted that the situation had "many parallels in etiological research, and cannot he held to constitute a material difficulty in attaining a connexion between the *Hecla* and the fever ashore."[26]

This was, in effect, a conclusion bearing upon the entire epidemic. Buchanan used it to generalize what local authorities had already concluded, namely, the *Hecla* posed a threat to public health. Action followed both decisions. Early suspicions of the ship had led municipal officials in Swansea to seek to isolate the *Hecla* from further human contacts and to proceed with disinfection.[27] Unloading being halted, her hatches were closed and she was disinfected with chlorine and thoroughly cleaned. On the twelfth unloading was renewed and by the twenty-first had been completed. All of this took place in response only to the case of Saunders; no other victim was identified as such until three deaths from yellow fever occurred on the twenty-second. A few days later, perhaps on the twenty-fourth or twenty-fifth, the *Hecla* was transferred to the Beaufort Dock (see map).

26. Ibid.
27. The treatment of the *Hecla* is described, ibid., pp. 453–454.

This at least removed the ship from public view; the Beaufort Dock was surrounded by tall warehouses.

On 27 September Buchanan reached Swansea. The following day he persuaded the reluctant Cobre agent to move the ship to the jetty in the outer harbor. The mayor of Swansea had constantly urged this step and popular opinion, Buchanan observed, was set on burning her at the dock that very evening were she not moved. Lashed to the jetty, the *Hecla* was unprotected against the elements and the nervous agent pleaded for her return to safety in the port. She was again disinfected and renewed appeals were made for readmission: that of 10 October was refused but permission was granted on the fourteenth. During this period the Cobre company, using a chlorine solution, disinfected the ore that had been unloaded from the *Hecla*, and the local board of health assured that all houses that had sheltered yellow-fever victims were fumigated with chlorine and then whitewashed.[28]

These measures approximate those applied to the *Anne-Marie*. In Swansea as in Saint-Nazaire, public recognition of the threat of a ship-related epidemic led first to hesitant isolation of the offending vessel within the port and then to her banishment from the port. In France the latter measure was but a preliminary to exacting cleansing and disinfection, inflicted by means of *sabordement* in the shallows on the opposite bank of the Loire; in Swansea the *Hecla* was treated in less radical manner. In both cases crewmen and, in the case of the *Hecla*, passengers had also dispersed before a full measure of the peril had been taken. But also in both cases, other persons — new susceptibles — were required to carry out the unloading of the ships and to conduct the maneuvers and cleansing operations that sound hygiene dictated. These latter parties were of great interest to Mélier but received scarcely a mention from Buchanan or Simon.

The Sanitarian's Solution

Buchanan acted in Swansea as the deputy of the Medical Officer of the Privy Council. This office had been created by the Public Health Act of 1858. The Medical Officer was charged with conducting inquiries into the public health and was required to bring his findings and his recommendations before the Council. At the outset there was no regular professional staff. Working only with part-time physician inspectors, John Simon

---

28. To London (and Swansea) observers, temperatures in Wales during the epidemic seemed truly "tropical," that is, they ranged steadily in the 70s and 80s F. There then followed a sharp break in temperature in early October. The connection, if any, between temperature changes and the end of the epidemic was not explored.

found his stated responsibility, to inquire and report, peculiarly congenial and he did both with a vengeance.

His training and experience in medicine were extensive. Educated in Germany and the London hospitals, Simon (1816–1904) was associated especially with St. Thomas's Hospital, serving as both surgeon and pathologist.[29] Beginning in 1848, he accepted the first in a succession of positions which placed him at the center of British public health work for some forty years. He served as Medical Officer to the City of London under the first Board of Health (1848–1854); Medical Officer to its successor, the General Board of Health (1855–1858); Medical Officer of the Privy Council, his most influential position (1858–1871); and, lastly, chief Medical Officer of the new Local Government Board (1871–1876). He then left regular public employment but remained active in various advisory capacities into the 1890s. His career literally embraced and, in many essential regards, constituted the great age of sanitary inquiry and the beginnings of British state medicine.

In all of these positions Simon exploited the power of information. He sought by means of private persuasion and incessant public discussion to influence both public opinion and state policy, confident that the former would help steer the latter. Simon's position represented the central government's concern and authority in the still ill-defined domain of public health. His agency was, in fact, in the later 1850s and 1860s, virtually the only central agency concerned with such medical matters. But powers of local inspection, and above all local action, rested with local boards of health and these bodies owed no allegiance to the Privy Council nor therefore to Simon. Until major changes were introduced under the Sanitary Act of 1866 — a turning point in the definition of permissible public sanitary intervention — the central government could exert little direct influence over the conduct of medical affairs on the local level, including control over access to ports in the British Isles.[30]

Great Britain in 1865 still lived under the quarantine law of 1825. This law allowed local authorities to control maritime traffic (though few, if any, did so) and gave no powers to the central government in these affairs. The latter might advise, but it could not initiate or intervene. Simon favored this arrangement. He also realized that the capacity to apply quarantine measures in Britain had very nearly reached its nadir. "I dare say,"

29. See the model biography by Royston Lambert, *Sir John Simon, 1816–1904, and English Social Administration* (London: MacGibbon and Kee, 1963).

30. Ibid., pp. 380–391, 395–399. Also Simon, *English Sanitary Institutions, Reviewed in the Course of their Development, and in Some of their Political and Social Relations* (London: Cassell, 1890; reprint, 1970), pp. 298–300.

he observed, "that quarantine in England was never otherwise than very lax. And at all events for many years past it has, in every medical sense, been abolished. Also with its virtual extinction, the establishment for giving it effect has declined. . . . the result of the entire process may be told in these very few words – that, at the present moment England [and also Wales] has not in readiness the means of properly quarantining even a single ship."[31] This was not cause for concern, because Britain would want to find a way to protect herself that would avoid the needless rigors of traditional quarantine.

Mélier's procedures in Saint-Nazaire, subsequently applied elsewhere in France, represented the formalization of a modified form of quarantine. These modifications had been introduced over several preceding generations; taken together, they reflected the abandonment of indiscriminate application of isolation measures to all components of an arrival – men, cargo, and ship. Earlier inflexibility was replaced by protective measures determined by the character of the disease and other factors determined to be relevant. Mélier insisted that men and women remain a part of this calculus. The observation and isolation of persons was essential to his plan, and port authorities were therefore obliged to create and maintain appropriate facilities. Here was a fundamental difference between French and British plans for national sanitary protection, between Mélier's solution and Simon's response to the yellow-fever problem: the former would control all aspects of an arrival, the latter permitted men and women to move freely into a port.

Simon used the epidemic in Swansea to develop general views on the question of quarantine. Some of these views had a basis in epidemiological experience, others quite obviously were a reflection of the mercantile mission of the British nation. The Privy Council's own physician announced:

A quarantine which is ineffective is a mere irrational derangement of commerce; and a quarantine, of the kind which ensures success, is more easily imagined than realized. Only in proportion as a community lives apart from the great highways and emporia of commerce, or is ready and able to treat its commerce as a subordinate political interest, only in such proportion can quarantine be made effectual for protecting it. In proportion as these circumstances are reversed, it becomes impossible to reduce to practice the paper plausibilities of quarantine. The conditions which have to be fulfilled of such conditions by England would involve fundamental changes in the most established habits of the country.[32]

31. Simon, "Yellow Fever at Swansea," p. 42.
32. Ibid., p. 41.

Given such conditions, and also given this outlook, it is not surprising that no provision was made or projected in Britain for the controlled observation of crew members, passengers, or workers who had been aboard an infected ship.

A second argument against quarantine was pragmatic: it simply did not work. Quarantine had not stopped the entry of Asiatic cholera into Britain and had worked no better on countless other occasions in countless other lands. Simon adopted an all-or-nothing view of the matter, confident that quarantine belonged in the latter category. To be effective, he demanded that quarantine be conducted with the "precision of a chemical experiment."[33] Quarantine required sustained and complete isolation of the sick and the suspect from all other members of society and also the separation of these two isolated parties from one another. Mélier's operations with hospital hulks and observations ships appeared to assure these conditions; Simon was confident that such arrangements could not be made in Britain. There was, furthermore, no way to be absolutely certain that all carriers of the disease had been discovered. Personal and commercial evasion was the rule wherever quarantine was imposed, and it only required one infectious person or one infected ship to destroy the entire edifice. And, for all of this inconsequential activity, the cost was very high: travel was seriously disrupted, trade was impeded, a merchant's quarantine costs could exceed the value of his cargo, and the public purse would be obliged to pay for all the usual inefficiencies of public administration. Here were reasons enough to refuse to use quarantine to defend the British Isles from continental or maritime epidemics. The fact is, Simon declared, that "contagions current on the continent of Europe must be deemed virtually current in England."[34]

At the Registrar General's office, William Farr, Britain's leading medical statistician and an accomplished epidemiologist, was no less blunt. When an inquiry regarding quarantine conducted by the National Association for the Promotion of Social Science turned to listing recommendations, these were stated to "amend and utilize, not to discontinue or to abolish the existing machinery" of quarantine. Farr, however, who had been an active member of the association's quarantine committee, immediately and disconcertingly announced that while he agreed with the conclusions of the report, he could not agree that "that introduction of dangerous dis-

33. Ibid., p. 40.
34. Ibid., p. 43. The challenge was also directed to the continuing British debate over central versus local government powers. Despite heavy pressure, Simon would not yield to the demand, raised especially by the cholera epidemic of 1866, to impose a centrally controlled national quarantine: see Lambert, *Sir John Simon*, pp. 377–380.

eases can be prevented by any quarantine regulations."[35] This was only to declare that the entire inquiry had been conducted on a false premise. Quarantine, however conducted, was worthless.

Now, this conclusion might seem obvious to anyone who claimed that yellow fever was a noncontagious disease. With such a disease the proper approach was disinfection, not the separation of persons, and this was the solution adopted by Simon. A sanitary attack on an offending object or objects would provide suitable protection. Such thoughts led Simon to ponder anew the confused world of contagionism and noncontagionism and loosely to gather epidemiological evidence from the Swansea epidemic that pertained to the question. His *Eighth Annual Report* to the Privy Council is a fascinating document in the evolution of disease theory, an unsteady portrait of the many possibilities and few certainties that marked the subject during the 1860s.

Simon placed typhoid fever and cholera in the contagious category alongside smallpox and syphilis.[36] In order to prevent the epidemic appearance of these contagious diseases, one might first think of trying to deny the causal principle access to a susceptible population. Quarantine was the measure designed for this purpose; however, it did not work. Viewing the matter from the sanitarian's perspective, Simon knew that the most effective counterattack had to be one that was launched from within. He and his associates on the Privy Council moved against contagion on the local level, using the well-tested measures of street cleaning, cesspool emptying, water purification, chemical disinfection, and the like. These were the primary weapons of the sanitary party and they had been brought to perfection, at least in theory, by English sanitarians of Simon's own generation and not least by Simon himself. Simon was no sanitary fanatic of the likes of Edwin Chadwick or his inflamed partisan, Florence Nightingale (one of whose principal bêtes noires was John Simon, a precarious position indeed).[37] To be sure, Simon's overall orientation was sanitary. He held that proper public-health administration had to deal first of all with the condition of environmental factors (water, food, housing, sewage, labor, and much else), but he tempered the exclusivities of this outlook with an open-mindedness to other possibilities. These included concern for the character of the causal agent or agents of communicable disease, an interest only to be expected of a pathologist.

But still a question remained, was yellow fever, too, a contagious dis-

35. William Farr, in "Report on Quarantine," *Parliamentary Papers* 58 (1861), p. 36.
36. Simon, "Yellow Fever at Swansea," p. 35n.
37. Lambert, *Sir John Simon*, pp. 267–269.

ease? This question simply would not vanish, even as Simon attempted to resolve the issue by verbal display.

> When phenomena of pestilence are under popular discussion and most of all when quarantine is being spoken of, frequently language is used which seems to imply a belief that the medical profession is divided as it were into two camps, respectively of 'contagionists' and 'anti-contagionists.' Now, so far as my knowledge extends, I venture to say (speaking of course of the medical profession as represented by its acknowledged teachers) that no such duality of opinion exists. . . . Ambiguities which fifty years ago existed in respect of some particular cases have since then been gradually cleared away. . . . More and more the once chaotic phenomenology of contagion is tending to become an intelligible and consistent section in the great science of organic chemistry.[38]

Simon's chemical theory of etiology was but another statement of the zymotic theory, derived from Justus von Liebig's theory of molecular excitation (see chapter 5). It served the useful purpose of moving the mind away from the divisive simplicities of contagionism and noncontagionism. It also indicates the possibility of an etiological middle ground, one which, however, was soon to be occupied by a living germ and not a particular chemical species.

Simon was unable to comply with his own rules of reasoning. Like so many others, he waded clumsily if assertively into the deep waters of etiological dispute. The critical question, again, was whether yellow fever could be transmitted directly from one person to another. The events at Saint-Nazaire, Dr. Chaillon notwithstanding, were ambiguous, so much so that contagion seemed an altogether incorrect conclusion to draw from them.

> But almost unquestionably, with regard to the *Anne-Marie,* and not improbably with regard to the *Chastan[g],* it seems that the ship, irrespectively of sick persons in it, was a focus of yellow fever infection. And, on this showing, the alleged facts admit of more than one interpretation. Whether, namely, the men carried infection because they themselves had contracted yellow fever, or merely carried infection passively as they might have carried an odour from the ship; whether men who had laboured in the hold of the *Anne-Marie* without themselves contracting yellow fever there might equally have carried infection to their homes; whether they who carried infection might have been disinfected by soap and water and change of dress; whether, in short, the infective power belonged, not to the sick body, as such, and to its excretions and discharges, but to the mere washable surface and clothing which had been saturated with the atmosphere of the ship; this question remains unanswered

38. Simon, "Yellow Fever at Swansea," p. 35.

by facts in the present record. And I draw attention to that openness of the question, because of its all-important bearing on the practical issue, whether it was necessary to adopt at Saint-Nazaire the system of personal quarantine which certain of M. Mélier's regulations enforced.[39]

This is disingenuous: Simon all too obviously trusted that his readers would conclude that yellow fever was not a contagious disease. After all, soap and water, the enthusiastic sanitarian's classic measures, could not reach and remedy a problem if the infective principle did in fact reside within and not on the surface of the sick individual.

Simon himself did not observe any of the events at Swansea and may never have seen a case of yellow fever, much less an epidemic of the disease. He consequently followed Buchanan's reasoning on the disputed matter of etiology. Certain cases at Swansea, the latter pointed out, could perhaps be explained by the movement of a specific contagion from one victim to another.[40] One household, for example, offered five victims, and another presented two cases. In these instances, personal contact was close and seemed to explain transmission of the disease. On the other hand, most of these victims, who resided on the island between the Tawe and the North Dock, could have been exposed to an infected atmosphere emanating from the hold or elsewhere aboard the *Hecla*. There was no way to distinguish between the rival causes. Furthermore, victims off-island might have been attacked not by some product of a diseased person's body but by part of an original, probably miasmatic cause traveling with that person. As noted above, Buchanan believed that this hypothesis might best explain the origin of the two most improbable cases, those of the Hickeys.

On the assumption that yellow fever was contagious, the distribution of the victims in Swansea and elsewhere should have created some twelve centers from which the disease then spread, the focus of each center being a sick individual. But not one person in the town "whose business did not lead [him or her] to the infected neighbourhood of the docks" contracted yellow fever. Surely the thousands of healthy innocents in Swansea were susceptible to the disease and there was no doubt that "many of the town's localities were perfectly adapted for the spread of contagious diseases." But the fact remained that in Swansea there was no hint whatsoever that the disease had spread, and from this fact Buchanan concluded that "if yellow fever was communicable at all by personal contagion it was so only

39. Ibid., p. 33.
40. Buchanan, "Report on Yellow Fever at Swansea," pp. 452–453. Simon's considered views on this subject appear in his article "Contagion" (1876), reprinted in John Simon, *Public Health Reports*, 2 vols., ed. Edward Seaton (London: Sanitary Institute, J. and A. Churchill, 1887), 2:561–585.

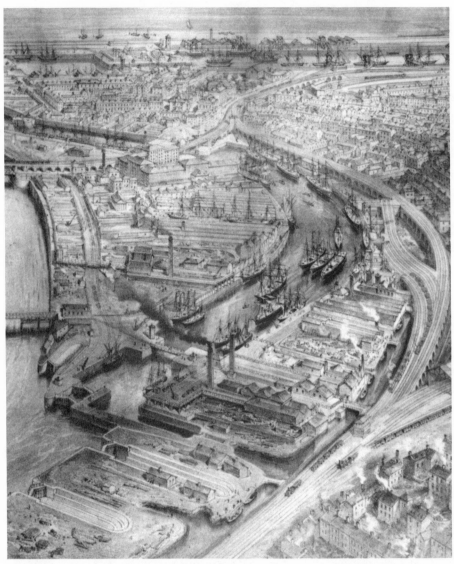

The North Dock at Swansea, ca. 1880. At the left, the river Tawe, and at the top (south)
the Bristol Channel. The *Hecla*, bearing copper ore and yellow fever, was moored in 1865
just off the apex of the curve midway along the North Dock. The large buildings above
middle center are the Beaufort Docks, within whose walls the *Hecla* was hidden when suspicions arose regarding that ship's sanitary condition. In the foreground is an indication of
the intensity of metallurgical activity in the Swansea region. (City of Swansea Archives,
Courtesy of the Swansea City Council.)

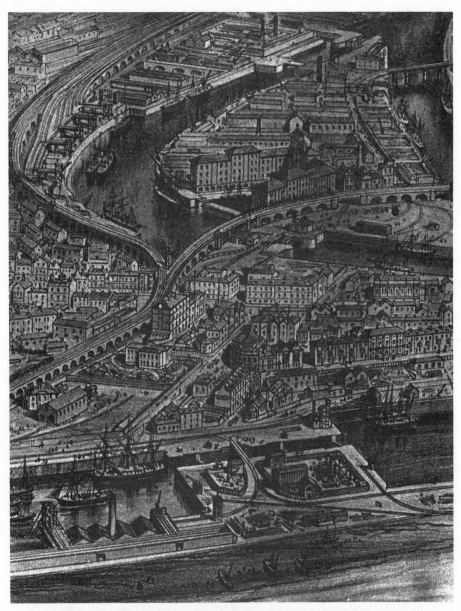

The North Dock seen from the south, ca. 1880. Below is the outer port and, above the viaduct, the Beaufort Dock. To the left, across the North Dock, railroad installations have replaced the housing where victims of the 1865 yellow-fever epidemic had lived; the Island between the North Dock and the Tawe was not, as can readily be seen, a major residential area. (City of Swansea Archives, Courtesy of the Swansea City Council.)

in an extremely feeble degree."[41] The fact that new cases of the disease, allowance being made for a period of incubation, stopped when the *Hecla* was removed from the harbor reaffirmed these negative arguments.

Obviously, one cannot turn to Buchanan and Simon, any more than to François Mélier, Nicolas Chervin, Wilhelm Griesinger, or the entire host of commentators on the yellow-fever phenomenon, for a definitive resolution of the etiology of the disease. In fact, Buchanan and Simon, although verging on the doctrinaire in their views, devoted no great part of their discussion to the matter. The principal task before the British inquirers was, as it had been in Saint-Nazaire, to decide upon appropriate protective measures. In this regard, etiology was suggestive, yet what proved decisive was not the causal question but the central epidemiological fact: yellow fever is an imported disease. This was recognized by both the French and the British observers.

Still, Simon found it difficult to move toward his goal. Etiological uncertainty made planning of hygienic action very awkward and Simon trimmed. One had to conclude, he admitted, that yellow fever might be both contagious and noncontagious. In short, confusion was his answer and caution his recommendation.

> I do not pretend to say that yellow fever is absolutely non-contagious in this country: non-contagious, I mean, in the sense in which typhus and smallpox are contagious: much less do I pretend to say that it is absolutely non-contagious in climates hotter than our own. . . . And though undoubtedly at St. Nazaire there were a few facts which led M. Mélier to impute contagiousness to the disease, the overwhelming majority of facts pointed, even there, to an opposite conclusion, and suggested that in the exceptional instances some source of fallacy had been overlooked. Quite unquestionable, however, is the evidence that the infection of yellow fever accompanies marine traffic from land to land; and in proportion as the belief is untenable that the disease is personally contagious, in such measure the alternative must be accepted — that infectiveness is truly in the body of the ship.[42]

In effect, noncontagionism was made the doctrinal residuum resulting from exclusion of the contagionist alternative. There was no proof that a particular miasma had caused a particular disease, but there seemed to be am-

41. Buchanan, "Report on Yellow Fever at Swansea," p. 453.

42. Simon, "Yellow Fever at Swansea," p. 45. Simon phrased his remarks as if they conveyed accepted opinion. But what persuaded Simon had not persuaded Mélier: the latter cited four possible cases of contagiousness, cast doubts on three but felt compelled to announce that the fourth (Alphonse Chaillon) confirmed that yellow fever was also a contagious disease. Simon in effect assigned his French colleague's interpretation of Chaillon's case to some kind of "fallacy," whether in evidence or argument not being indicated.

ple evidence that that cause was not a discrete contagion. This, of course, had long been and remained a central argument of the British sanitary party and of noncontagionists everywhere.

Simon could now use his conclusion to articulate a course of action. If a particular miasma, a given noncontagion, had not been captured and dissected, as indeed it had not, still its existence seemed undeniable and, what was of supreme importance, its behavior displayed its weak points. In a summary presentation of his views, Simon declared that

> yellow fever is a malarious rather than a truly zymotic disease, is a disease of the nature of ague rather than a disease of the nature of typhus,— that the ship which spreads infection does so irrespectively of the persons who are in it, whether they be healthy or diseased,— that the ferment of a local and impersonal infection clings to the ship from shore to shore, and breeds new malarious action in any congenial soil to which it comes,— that the exceptional and contingent powers of persons to spread the disease is generally but a very scanty and transient power, not belonging particularly to the sick, but to the healthy in common with them, attaching perhaps mainly to their dress, and equally predicable of all absorbent things which the atmosphere of the ship has imbued; — this, it seems to me, is the doctrine of yellow fever which tallies best with our present knowledge of facts.[43]

There is much in this statement that might receive comment but only one point requires emphasis here. Simon accepted the notion of the importation of yellow fever and agreed, too, that this disease is a "local and impersonal infection." But with regard to the origin of the infection, "local" referred to some other locality; yellow fever had not been produced *de novo* from the soil of Swansea or, for that matter, from local conditions elsewhere in Europe. It is precisely this conclusion that separates Simon and Buchanan—as well as Mélier, who reasoned no differently—from traditional noncontagionist understanding. The latter would have an apparently exotic disease such as yellow fever arise from a singular conjunction of local conditions, "local" now assuredly embracing Britain and the European continent. The former had no solution to the riddle of origins but believed that they had solved the problem of the occurrence of yellow fever in Europe: it was introduced from abroad.

Simon concluded that what had checked the epidemic in Saint-Nazaire, that is, prevented the further spread of yellow fever, was not the detention of persons who had disembarked from or had had contact with the *Anne-Marie*. It was, instead, Mélier's sanitary assault on that ship and continued action by others addressed to later arrivals. From this perspective the

43. Ibid., pp. 45–46.

quarantine problem simply disappeared of its own accord. There need be no delay upon arrival save for the quickly handled routine of cleansing and disinfection. No heroic measures such as *sabordement* or a massive hygienic attack were required; one needed only purify the air aboard a ship and rid her of potential sources of renewed infection such as bilge water, dirty clothing, or fouled latrines. Persons need not be detained.

British law, however, did not make this an easy matter, for one was, after all, intending to interfere directly with private property. Simon, who never failed in ingenious extension of the law, solved the problem literally by claiming new territory for Britain. He announced that "ships coming into port and thus annexing themselves to inhabited territory" fell subject to the powers of local port authorities.[44] They were to be subject, therefore, to the provisions of the Nuisances Removal and Diseases Prevention Acts of 1855 and the modifications made to them in 1860. In those cases where local authorities took action on their own volition or could be prodded into action by the Privy Council's Medical Officer, a sanitary defense could be mounted. The former was the case at Swansea, local initiative receiving subsequent support from Buchanan and Simon. As described earlier, the *Hecla* was cleaned, disinfected, and isolated—actions undertaken by the Cobre Association under pressure from the municipality.

There was one further argument against quarantine and against those who might be tempted to consider its revival. Simon offered a strange combination in which theoretical inappropriateness and satisfying public incapacity conspired to destroy any thought of erecting major barriers against yellow fever. Quarantine was intended to prevent the entrance of a communicable disease amidst a susceptible population. Contagionists insisted that quarantine control the movement of men and women as well as that of ships and cargo; noncontagionists held that the human body posed little or no threat to the public health. It seemed reasonable to Simon to contemplate that quarantine measures used to prevent entry of a genuine contagious disease might be applied also to yellow fever. Although the latter was not demonstrably contagious and in fact seemed not to be contagious at all, Simon was willing, argumentatively at least, to reduce an already slight risk even further by acting as if the disease could be contagious. This seemed sound caution; in truth, it was absurd. Should Britain, he asked, presume to introduce quarantine against a disease which at most was doubtfully contagious, when it faced a host of other diseases that were notori-

44. Simon, "Remarks by the Medical Officer of the Privy Council" [on the Regulations made by the French Government, with the Advice of M. Mélier (1861)], *Parliamentary Papers* 33 (1866) [note 1, above], p. 474. See Lambert, *Sir John Simon*, pp. 321–322.

ously contagious and against which it presented no defenses at all? Britain made no effort to halt the introduction of smallpox or typhus fever, both contagious diseases in Simon's opinion. Why, then, be so foolish as to begin with yellow fever? This would be only "to precautionize in the inverse ratio of our actual experiences of danger."[45]

Swansea and Saint-Nazaire

Yellow fever at Swansea led Buchanan and Simon to conclusions very similar to those reached earlier by Mélier. Yellow fever was an imported disease. Its point of entry at Swansea was the North Dock and its vehicle the *Hecla;* at Saint-Nazaire, its point of entry was the Quai Jégou and it had been borne by the *Anne-Marie.* In both cases the disease was not a local product. Moreover, the disease in question was a specific disease, a definite clinical entity not to be confounded with or derived from other diseases.

With regard to etiology, Buchanan, Simon, and Mélier were essentially noncontagionists. All three broke, however, with earlier noncontagionist doctrine regarding yellow fever and refused to accept the notion that strictly local conditions could generate this disease. The idea of specificity and the evidence favoring importation weighed overwhelmingly against the local origins hypothesis. Noncontagionism and local origins, the inseparable core concepts of yellow-fever theory from the 1820s into the 1850s, were thus disjoined, and the latter was categorically denied.

The parallel between British and French understanding of the disease and its control reaches somewhat further, but there are also differences between these viewpoints—significant differences based upon both disease theory and experience with or expectations of respective national administrative practice. Mélier preferred a conservative understanding of the movement of yellow fever: if person-to-person transmission was a possibility, however rare that event be, then appropriate protective measures had to be devised and introduced. This entailed close attention to the length of the incubation period of yellow fever and regular imposition, whenever suspicions were aroused, of a set period of observation (or provision of care) for persons arriving aboard an infected vessel. Simon, however, came very close to exonerating crewman and passenger; he reserved his attentions for cargo and, above all, for the ship—neither of which, of course, was overlooked by Mélier. In Simon's view, an attack was to be launched with ease and efficacy against, literally, the surface of things—against those

45. Simon, "Remarks by the Medical Officer of the Privy Council," p. 474.

objects (the human skin, clothing, luggage, fomites of all kinds, and cased or loose cargo) with which the infective miasma had had an opportunity to make contact.

Still, Simon felt compelled to have it both ways, and then to back away again. He recalled that in Britain one approach, modified quarantine of persons, was unattainable in practice and therefore required no further consideration. He admitted that the contagionist hypothesis, if applied to yellow fever, would authorize a period of observation, acknowledging that the length of this period would be determined by the incubation period assigned to the disease. He was quite skeptical, however, of Mélier's estimate of this period, especially its lesser limit (three days), and implied that the incubation period of yellow fever would usually be considerably longer or at least extremely variable.[46] All of this suggested anew the vanity of any effort to quarantine persons, a vanity which Simon saw reflected in the utter absence in Britain of facilities with which to conduct such a quarantine. He reasoned less accurately, however, when he attempted to transfer his own doubts to Mélier, suggesting that Mélier, too, had reasoned in an expedient and not a rigorous manner.[47]

Neither Buchanan and Simon nor Mélier had the least clue as to the character of the presumed causal agent of the disease. The former spoke freely of a definite "zymotic" agent but possessed no empirical substance to attach to that label; Mélier's unknown "principle" of yellow fever offered nothing more. All three observers proceeded on the assumption of the existence of such a causal agent, and each drew conclusions consistent with what were deemed essential attributes of this agent, namely, its specificity and capacity to move in or as a miasma. What had authorized this characterization of the disease agent? Its attributes had been derived not from study of the agent per se, from etiological inquiry in a strict sense, but represented only deductions from the epidemic behavior of yellow fever. Virtually all that was learned at Swansea and Saint-Nazaire regarding the nature and behavior of yellow fever was obtained by strictly epidemiological inquiry. Probably no single discovery made during these investigations constituted new knowledge. The complicated behavior of the disease had been closely observed for some one hundred and fifty years. But Buchanan and Simon and, especially, Mélier went further and were favored by unusual circumstances. Their northern epidemics provided a quasi-

46. Ibid., pp. 471–472.

47. "If M. Mélier had not framed his regulations on a contagionistic basis, he might indeed have been praised by noncontagionists for omitting superfluous precautions, but (especially after the startling fact of M. Chaillon's death) could scarcely have hoped to satisfy the local population that he had advised every desirable precaution." Ibid., p. 472.

controlled observational field and permitted the exhaustive and exact de-
lineation of the course and conditions of discrete epidemic events.

Of decisive importance for their accomplishment was the careful use
of case-tracing, a method inseparable from the combined notions of a discrete disease moving in a definite manner. Buchanan and Simon shared
with Mélier a new faith, perhaps the most important contribution of early
epidemiology to the investigation of and efforts to control communicable
disease. This was the idea of the epidemiological distinctiveness of each
such disease. The recurrent epidemics of the mid-nineteenth century had
provided a powerful stimulus to such thinking. Endemic diseases, such as
typhoid fever, acquired thereby a new set of defining parameters, epidemic
behavior being added to pathological anatomy and clinical description;
and exotic diseases, whose most frequent representative was Asiatic cholera, received even more exacting and abundant attention from a sizable
army of investigators. The epidemics at Saint-Nazaire and at Swansea allowed yellow fever to be brought within the reach of such thinking.

III

What Was Epidemiology?

7

What Was Epidemiology?

DEFINITION IS a difficult and uncertain art, and a definition of epidemiology is not easily obtained. Epidemiology emerged as a self-conscious science during the 1840s, yet it did so without a single, clearly formulated or widely accepted goal and without an assured sense of the methods the science should employ. Since that time, however, there has been a discernible direction to the evolution of both definition and epidemiological concern. The beginnings of epidemiology as a recognized science were firmly planted in the description and assessment of the historical and geographical parameters of communicable disease. The epidemiologist sought to determine the reasons for the occurrence of epidemics and of the single epidemic. He did so by ascertaining the historical, spatial, and temporal conditions of an epidemic. The dominant effort in epidemiological inquiry was exploration of the local conditions that favored or hindered that epidemic. Epidemiological interpretation then framed its explanations in environmentalist terms — that is, explanatory precedence was assigned to the morbific influence of climatic or atmospheric factors.

After 1880, however, this focus was replaced by the lessons taught by the germ theory of disease. An all-encompassing biomedical orientation now entered epidemiology. Increasingly, emphasis was placed on the character and behavior of the infective agent of disease (usually a microorganism) and on the pathogenic activity of this agent. Environmental conditions were not forgotten, but their role in epidemiological investigation and explanation was greatly reduced. With surprising rapidity, epidemiology became and long remained the "science of the infective diseases — their prime causes, propagation, and prevention. More especially it deals with their epidemic manifestations. . . . Infective disease . . . is a process, namely the specific interaction of specific microbic parasites and of host." Most recent generations continue this emphasis but also stress that population phenomena of all kinds should also be among the epidemiologist's preoccupations.

This definitional quest has not slackened. Some have found the distinctiveness and purpose of epidemiology in the epistemological domain. Epidemiology thus becomes a sophisticated form of "problem solving." Moreover, while preserving its traditional connection with the infectious diseases, epidemiology now embraces chronic disease as well. One might best view epidemiology as "a way of learning, of asking questions and getting answers that lead to further questions." A recent definition embraces virtually all of these tendencies: "Epidemiology can be regarded as a sequence of reasoning concerned with biological inferences derived from observations of disease occurrence and related phenomena in human population groups."[1]

These definitions all reflect twentieth-century understanding and draw confidence and orientation from the bases established by the germ theory. Physicians before 1880 lacked this confidence. Although epidemiology in the 1850s and 1860s did seek disciplinary awareness, and programmatic statements were already numerous, it is striking how few of those who engaged in exacting empirical work attempted to give general definition to their enterprise. John Snow, whose studies of the London cholera epidemics of the 1840s and 1850s have rendered his one of the most celebrated names in the history of the science, scarcely expressed himself on the nature of epidemiology (his principal medical concern was, in fact, anesthesiology). John Simon did little more. Even Max von Pettenkofer, the most influential epidemiologist of the mid-nineteenth century and another ardent student of epidemic cholera, rarely ventured comment on the nature of his science. It is not surprising, therefore, that neither François Mélier nor George Buchanan made an attempt to define the limits of epidemiology.

The need to do so, however, was real and was not unrecognized. Acting upon the request of his colleagues in the British Medical Association, William Budd attempted to provide an outline of the principal features of epidemiological reasoning. He, too, was an accomplished epidemiologist, perhaps the most imaginative and insistent inquirer of his generation. He was able to create a portrait of his science by assembling in roughly reasoned form the basic rubrics under which epidemiological inquiry had been and, Budd believed, was henceforth to be conducted. Budd's views are further interesting because of the overt etiological bias that informed his discussion; epidemiology without etiology, indeed, without the contagionist interpretation of causation, seemed to him quite inconceivable.

Budd's position, however, also serves to define more clearly the char-

1. For these various definitions, see C. O. Stallybrass, *The Principles of Epidemiology and the Process of Infection* (London: Macmillan, 1931), pp. v, 27; J. P. Fox et al., *Epidemiology. Man and Disease* (New York: Macmillan, 1970), p. v; J. N. Morris, *Uses of Epidemiology* (London: Churchill, Livingstone, 1975), p. 3; A. M. Lilienfeld and D. E. Lilienfeld, *Foundations of Epidemiology* (New York: Oxford University Press, 1980), p. 4. See D. E. Lilienfeld, "Definitions of Epidemiology," *American Journal of Epidemiology* 107 (1978): 87–90; R. R. Frerichs and Raymond Neutra, "Letter to the Editor," ibid., 108 (1978): 74–75.

acter of epidemiology at a time when that science was pursued without a reliable solution to the causal question. In this form, epidemiology was essentially the study of disease transmission, and careful case-tracing was its most effective means of investigation. Case-tracing immediately raises the crucial question of the circumstances surrounding the first or early case or cases of an epidemic disease. Thus, in responding to the question, what was epidemiology?, I first use Budd's categories to describe the general features of the science, including the always ambiguous matter of etiology; I then set forth more fully the central importance of the first-case phenomenon.

But epidemiology in the mid-nineteenth century offers more than this. Writers on the history of the science have long recognized that epidemiology has important social and economic connections and was informed, particularly between 1820 and 1860, by strong ideological commitments. These latter bring into striking conjunction liberal political values, the centrality or even priority of environmental (atmospheric) disease causation, and an issue fundamental to all public health discussion and activity: the nature, possibility, and desirability of scientific control over major features of the human condition. Atmospheric causation, it seemed, presupposed and perpetuated social distance at the same time that it provided a basis for scientific intervention into human affairs. Social distance reflected a dominant political stance and thus science appeared to provide an additional foundation for assuring the socioeconomic status quo. In my concluding section, I offer further if brief comment on these themes, drawing upon the lessons taught by the yellow-fever epidemics and investigations described in this book.

The Dimensions of Epidemiology

William Budd's interest in epidemiology had begun in the 1830s, and it continued undiminished throughout long years of medical practice. Born in Devonshire, Budd (1811–1880) received an excellent medical education and then entered practice in Bristol and in the west of England. He acquired there exceptional experience with communicable diseases and was highly regarded in the profession for his study of their distribution and behavior.[2] His most important epidemiological studies dealt with typhoid

2. E. W. Goodall, *William Budd: M.D. Edin., F.R.S. The Bristol Physician and Epidemiologist* (Bristol: Arrowsmith, 1936); Margaret Pelling, *Cholera, Fever and English Medicine, 1825–1865* (Oxford: Oxford University Press, 1978), pp. 146–202, 250–294; Editor's "Foreword" and "Afterword" in William Budd, *On the Causes of Fever. On the Causes and Mode of Propagation of the Common Continued Fevers of Great Britain and Ireland,* ed. D. C. Smith (Baltimore: Johns Hopkins University Press, 1984).

fever in the rural and urban setting and with the spread of Asiatic cholera during the second and third British outbreaks of this disease (1848–1849; 1853–1854). Budd was convinced that the progress of epidemiology depended upon understanding the mode of propagation of the demonstrably "contagious or communicable diseases." These diseases, notably smallpox, typhoid fever, and Asiatic cholera, were "open to more definite conclusions than can be come to as to the rest."[3] By 1849, and probably earlier, the idea of contagion had become in Budd's mind less a conclusion founded upon rigorous inquiry than the very premise of his investigations. He spoke of "contagion . . . as signifying the communication of a specific disease, through whatever medium, by specific germs thrown off by subjects already suffering from it."[4] Budd's epidemiology, obviously, was closely tied to etiology.

Mélier and Buchanan did not ignore the causal question and Nicolas Chervin was quite consumed by it. The former, however, regarded etiology as an important but inaccessible matter; this was altogether true of the yellow-fever epidemics of the 1860s. Budd followed a different route. He persuaded himself that the fundamental trait of all epidemic disease was its contagiousness. Hence, he insisted on determining not only the communicability of a disease, if in fact it proved to be communicable, but with equal dedication he attempted to discover that which was actually communicated. He ended by postulating what must be the properties of the (presumably living) agent that was transmitted between persons. Of course, these were properties of an agent which itself had not been apprehended. Budd had many plausible, even persuasive reasons for his view, but he also lived on faith. While this is a matter worthy of attention, and Budd did not stand alone, for present purposes it is sufficient to notice only that he steered his course by the etiological star. Mélier and Buchanan, being either less bold or more prudent, adopted a more phenomenological view of this tempting but very difficult problem of cause.

In seeking first principles for his science, Budd proceeded by interrogation. He posed a set of questions for the epidemiologist, the replies to which then defined the specific epidemiological character of a given communicable disease. These questions also framed the basic categories for epidemiological reasoning regarding any communicable disease. Budd's questions may be placed in three broad categories. These include (1) the behavior of the affected individual and the human disease process, (2) the relation between external conditions and individual or population propensity to

3. William Budd, "Investigation of Epidemic and Epizootic Diseases," *British Medical Journal* 2 (1864): 355.
4. William Budd, "Variola Ovina, Sheep's Smallpox; or the Laws of Contagious Epidemics Illustrated by an Experimental Type," *British Medical Journal* 2 (1863): 143n.

illness, and (3) population phenomena per se.[5] In the first category stood the general question of contagiousness, how the causal agent entered the body, the presence or absence of characteristic eruptions or excreta, incubation period, whether an attack confers lasting immunity, the role of the individual resistance of the host and of the virulence of the causal agent, and the decisive question of whether the induced disease is truly a specific entity or whether communicable diseases might, as some noncontagionists continued to claim, change one into another during the course of a severe epidemic. Under the heading of external conditions, Budd directed inquiries to the possible susceptibility of animals to human disease, what measures might be adopted to bring contagion to a halt, and what influence environmental conditions (climate, atmosphere, soil, and the like) exert. Here, too, belonged a question of great importance to all of Budd's reasoning and a proposition that he resolutely opposed: the spontaneous generation of pathogenic agents. Matters relating to population included the question as to when and where the first case or cases occurred, the geographical limits of the outbreak, what medium might be capable of spreading the disease, when virulence begins and when it ends (that is, what are the limits of infectivity in a population), and what proportion of cases can be connected with previous cases and what proportion cannot. Budd indicated by his emphases that population phenomena and external influences, although important, were not the foremost concern of the epidemiologist; contagion was.

Budd's essays on typhoid fever and cholera were as much medical as they were epidemiological reports.[6] They were the product of keen observation carried out in the course of medical practice. With regard especially to typhoid fever, Budd was determined to demonstrate the clinical unity of the disease and its pathological distinctness as this was reflected by characteristic intestinal lesions, and then to use both of these conclusions to further a third and perhaps the principal point, the contagiousness of typhoid fever. Epidemiological evidence and argument furthered this purpose and did not constitute an end in themselves. Despite his great interest and skill in epidemiological analysis, Budd did not provide a detailed portrait of the course of any epidemic.

On the subject of contagion, he was categorical: "Occurring, for the most part, under the eye of a single observer, and open to no ambiguity from any quarter," the several facts that he observed in the town of North Tawton and that pertained to epidemic typhoid fever "fulfill every condition that can be required of evidence in such a case; and, in spite of all

5. Budd, "Investigation of Epidemic and Epizootic Diseases," p. 355.
6. See references in Goodall, *William Budd*, pp. 145–147.

that has been asserted, and is still maintained, to the contrary, in high places, prove beyond question that this fever is an essentially contagious fever. If need were, it would be easy to show, by the severe logic of mathematical deduction, that to attempt to explain them on any other principle would not only be absurd, but outrageously so."[7] This view, a truly radical contagionist interpretation, reached far and was made to extend even further.

The results could be most unfortunate, but they illustrate well the peculiarly awkward place occupied by yellow fever in a discussion of epidemiological principles that drew its guidance from etiology. Budd was prey to hasty and startling conclusions regarding the transmission of this exotic disease.

> Whenever a contagious disorder is attended by discharges that are characteristic of it, these discharges are always . . . the chief vehicle of the morbid poison. They originate, in fact, in, and are the outward mark of, the very act of elimination. It is from this intimate connection with the specific poison, in each particular case, that such discharges derive their special character. I need scarcely add that yellow fever offers no exceptions to this law. [There is ample] evidence by which it may be shown that the black vomit and the secretions of the same kind which issue from the bowel have a very large if not principal part in the propagation of this pestilence. It may be sufficient to state here, that this conclusion may be deduced with the utmost certainty from already existing data.[8]

It followed that protection was readily available: one need only disinfect the vomit and feces of the yellow-fever victim. Too obviously, Budd had merely transferred to a new and to him unfamiliar disease explanatory principles and remedial measures that had proved appropriate to very different diseases. He thus transgressed against an important and new epidemiological rule, that which stated that distinct communicable diseases behave each in a distinct epidemiological manner.

Budd's roster of the major concerns of epidemiology virtually exhausted the preoccupations of the science. His special perspective did not, of course, grant all interests equal representation. Contagion dominated his arguments, and its epidemiological concomitant, the smallpox analogy, which had been expanded to embrace water-borne fevers, was improperly allowed to di-

---

7. Budd, "Intestinal Fever Essentially Contagious," *Lancet* 1 (1859): 55.

8. William Budd, "On the Contagion of Yellow Fever," *Lancet* 1 (1861): 337; see Pelling, *Cholera, Fever and English Medicine*, p. 252. John Snow also favored a water-borne cause of yellow fever: *On the Mode of Communication of Cholera* (London: John Churchill, 1855; reprinted as *Snow on Cholera, being a Reprint of Two Papers by John Snow, M.D., Together with a Biographical Memoir by B. W. Richardson, M.D.*, Introduction by W. H. Frost [New York: The Commonwealth Fund, 1936; reprint 1965]), p. 127.

rect inquiry into other communicable diseases such as yellow fever. Budd, in fact, was obsessed by unifactorial causation and viewed epidemiology as an instrument not for testing but for establishing the correctness of the contagion hypothesis.

But there were others who, although not uninterested in contested etiological matters, pursued epidemiological inquiries without presupposing or requiring a definitive answer to the question of causation. Mélier, Buchanan, and numerous others during the 1850s and 1860s, placed primary emphasis upon the question of transmission. Their theory asked what the pathways of disease transmission were; their action demanded to know what the most effective means of interrupting transmission were. The investigations at Saint-Nazaire and Swansea addressed precisely these questions. Mélier and Buchanan weighed the question of disease specificity and answered it in the affirmative: yellow fever was a distinct communicable disease and was not to be confused with or derived from a prevailing local infection. First and subsequent cases were identified and the relation of each case to others was clarified. It was immediately apparent that the disease in question was not an indigenous product and had, in fact, been introduced. Case-tracing, joined to exhaustive analysis of relevant local environmental conditions, thus eliminated the possibility of an endemic source of the disease and identified the only remaining source, namely, an infected ship arriving from an infected foreign port. The pursuit of this information was conducted in a thorough, careful, and timely manner, with the result that it was possible to reconstruct the sequence of epidemic events in Saint-Nazaire and in Swansea in a singularly complete and exact manner. Incubation period and immunity were also investigated, and the possibility of nonhuman hosts was explored and rejected.

This work illustrates well the several activities that Budd had included in his roster of the attributes of epidemiology. It deserves note, however, that Mélier and Buchanan emphasized the analysis of the relation between external conditions and the fate of affected individuals and offered consideration of limited aspects of population phenomena. These were the second and third domains of Budd's epidemiological principles; as remarked earlier, Budd stressed the importance of the first domain wherein etiology occupied pride of place.

It may be noted that neither Mélier nor Buchanan (nor Budd) made serious use of a new and promising tool for analyzing population phenomena, namely, statistics. The numbers they presented offered only a summary statement of the sick and the dead and were not further exploited. By 1860, the statistical ideal had been clearly stated and, in certain situations, put to effective use. Asiatic cholera proved to be the statistical disease par excellence, a function of its high mortality and conspicuous urban onslaughts; both Snow and von Pettenkofer established their reputations as epidemiologists by means of imaginative analyses of the movement of cholera in large cities.[9] Students of small epidemics, for obvious reasons, rarely followed this lead.

A final and now familiar dimension of epidemiology also deserves further attention. The specificity of communicable disease is the foundation of all rigorous epidemiological investigation. In the years around 1800, yellow fever provided no useful example, for the fact is that this disease was made a coherent medical entity only under the stimulus of analysis of other communicable diseases. As has been seen, Nicolas Chervin gathered together a set of tropical and temperate-zone fevers and called what he deemed to be the most severe form "yellow fever." The latter was not a distinct disease but only the extreme limit of a series of serious or less-serious fevers. Yellow fever could appear abruptly in localities in which the disease had not previously been encountered. It arose there from the heightening of local and less malignant fevers, the transformation being, apparently, the outcome of an interaction between changed local conditions and the intensity of the prevailing epidemic.

Chervin's view posed a serious difficulty, but one that has received little attention. Somehow a reliable criterion had to be devised for determining when sickness at large ceased being a common fever and became the serious affair known as yellow fever. Neither Chervin nor anyone else could begin to provide such a measure. What was true for collective illness would also be true for a few identifiable sick individuals and for the single in-

---

9. See Snow, *On the Mode of Communication of Cholera*; P. E. Brown, "John Snow — The Autumn Loiterer," *Bulletin of the History of Medicine* 35 (1961): 519–528; idem, "Another Look at John Snow," *Anesthesia and Analgesia: Current Researches* 43 (1964): 646–654; Lord Cohen of Birkenhead, "John Snow — The Autumn Loiterer?," *Proceedings of the Royal Society of Medicine* 62 (1969): 99–106. Also Max von Pettenkofer, "Ueber die Verbreitungsart der Cholera," *Zeitschrift für Biologie* 1 (1865): 322–374; *Ueber den gegenwärtigen Stand der Cholera-Frage und über die nächsten Aufgaben zur weiteren Ergründung ihrer Ursachen* (Munich: Oldenbourg, 1873); Wilhelm Rimpau, *Die Entstehung von Pettenkofers Bodentheorie und die Münchener Choleraepidemie von 1854. Eine kritisch-historische Studie.* Veröffentlichungen aus dem Gebiete der Medizinalverwaltung, Bd. 44, H. 7 (Berlin: Richard Schoetz, 1935); Karl Kisskalt, *Max von Pettenkofer* (Stuttgart: Wissenschaftliche Verlagsgesellschaft, 1948). See also A. M. Lilienfeld and D. E. Lilienfeld, "The Epidemiologic Fabric: Weaving the Threads, I., Weaving the Threads, II: The London Bridge — It Never Fell," *International Journal of Epidemiology* 9 (1980): 199–206, 299–304; J. M. Eyler, "William Farr on the Cholera: The Sanitarian's Disease Theory and the Statistician's Method," *Journal of the History of Medicine* 28 (1973): 79–100; idem, *Victorian Social Medicine. The Ideas and Methods of William Farr* (Baltimore: Johns Hopkins University Press, 1979), pp. 37–96, 159–201; and V. L. Hilts, "Epidemiology and the Statistical Movement," in *Times, Places and Persons. Aspects of the History of Epidemiology,* ed. A. M. Lilienfeld (Baltimore: Johns Hopkins University Press, 1980), pp. 43–55.

dividual; at some point, yellow fever *strictu sensu* would have to make its appearance. One might even ask, where did such a change occur: in a single sick individual? from one individual to the next? between a group of individuals and an immediately succeeding group? At what point during the course of an epidemic did this change take place, and why? There was no way to make sense of the problems that these questions, posed by hindsight, raise. Naturally, it was not difficult to *state* that a particular epidemic had begun with a relatively benign fever and had then revealed the face of yellow fever. Precisely this had occurred at Gibraltar, but members of the French commission had had no experience at all with the early stages of the epidemic and therefore could not speak authoritatively of the evolution (if any) of the disease itself. Neither this hindrance nor others, however, stopped Chervin from continuing to propagate his view.

Although dealing with a different communicable disease, Budd had seen clearly what was at stake when he defended so vigorously the unity of typhoid fever. He believed firmly that this conclusion followed without possibility of contradiction from repeated and exact observation of sick individuals. More important, he understood that this assurance and this assurance alone authorized an epidemiologist to follow the movement of "a" disease and to attempt to draw meaningful conclusions regarding an epidemic of "this" disease. Budd's whole outlook offered a categorical rejection of the ambitious notion of a multiform *gastroentérite* that had been announced by P. J. B. Broussais. Broussais's view had attained remarkably wide influence between 1815 and 1830, but his collection of gastrointestinal (and other) complaints into one diagnostic unit of disease directly opposed the activity of his contemporaries. Many of them were seeking to use pathological anatomy and careful clinical observation to distinguish specific disease entities and to determine the characteristic features of each.[10]

With precisely the same outlook, but perhaps without Budd's prophetic style, Mélier proceeded to analyze yellow fever. In agreement with other physicians, he discarded Chervin's protean notion of the disease. Yellow fever was a distinct disease; it was not to be confounded with or allowed to evolve from or into another fever. Individual cases of yellow fever could thus be confidently identified, and the connection of each with another case or with relevant environmental conditions could be specified. Pertinent external factors (a ship from a tropical port, for example) could also be identified and new, highly suggestive connections established. It is important to note that this kind of epidemiological inquiry is impossible without a well-founded confidence in the specificity of the disease under investiga-

10. See E. H. Ackerknecht, "Broussais, Or A Forgotten Medical Revolution," *Bulletin of the History of Medicine* 27 (1953): 320–343.

tion, or without appropriate circumscription of local conditions thought to be epidemiologically significant.

The First-Case Phenomenon

In epidemiology, factors such as geographical location, population and economic activity may be regarded as intrinsic to the epidemic itself. But communications and the timing and organization of an inquiry are generally under the control of the investigator. The problem common to all investigations is to translate the well-understood need for a critical, epidemiological outlook into the tangible realities of a specific investigation. Gibraltar, it appeared, offered great advantages. Yet here, in this isolated, none-too-populous community, these opportunities were utterly lost, largely because of disagreements as to the nature of the disease. Was it, physicians asked, truly yellow fever? Even if it was, was it not probable that this "new" disease was really only the malignant form of an endemic disease? If so, was it meaningful to speak of a first case of a disease whose very identity was in question? Indeed, how would one know a first case should one chance to meet it? The fact that the course of the Gibraltar epidemic was not exhaustively and precisely recorded only compounded these difficulties.

In contrast, at Saint-Nazaire and Swansea authentic data were assembled that represented virtually the entirety of the epidemic. The data were authentic not because they reflected with absolute accuracy the events that occurred, but because the information assembled was the product of observations made by physicians who set about their task with due deliberation and clear purpose. They were present when the events took place, surveyed the epidemic scene as completely as possible and ran careful checks on their own observations and on those made by associates. That most pregnant of epidemiological explanations — the conditions surrounding an epidemic — was, at Saint-Nazaire and to a lesser degree at Swansea, dissected, and the condition of each condition was recorded and evaluated. One such condition was identification in each of the two epidemics of the initial case or cases of yellow fever; the identification of these cases depended upon the early presence of alert and experienced observers.

The first-case phenomenon was a matter of keen interest in the early years of epidemiology. Budd, of course, recognized its great importance, giving the question a prominent place among his basic epidemiological propositions. French physicians were no less concerned. Armand Trousseau, an old hand in dealing with epidemic typhoid fever and cholera, as well as a member of the yellow-fever commission sent to Gibraltar (see chapter 2), always entertained little hope of getting to the bottom of an epidemic outbreak in an urban setting. In words that recall the views of Esprit Gendron quoted in chapter 1, he informed his students that "in Paris, as in all large population centers, we lack the information that we need to take us back to the origin of the troubles; we cannot arrive at a solution to such a complex problem. This solution, however, we have received from physicians who practice in small localities where one can easily [sic] discover the person who first became ill."[11] Ironically, however, it was in England and in a setting altogether contrary to Gendron's and Trousseau's expectations that the first-case phenomenon was given thorough consideration.

At the request of the General Board of Health, Edmund A. Parkes (1819–1876), by the middle 1840s an assistant physician in a London hospital and later one of Britain's leading hygienists (Professor of Hygiene, Army Medical School, first at Chatham, then at Netley), undertook to assess the matter of first cases. The Board of Health had been created by Parliament in 1848. Led by Edwin Chadwick between 1849 and 1855, it became the great engine of English hygienic investigation and action. To Chadwick and his associates no event was as exciting and no challenge as great as a large epidemic. As it had been for Snow and Budd, so it was for the Board of Health; the cholera epidemic of 1848–1849 created a host of promising investigative and interpretive possibilities.

Parkes's participation in these inquiries gave him abundant experience with cholera, and it provides us with a remarkable instance of the growing recognition that the conditions surrounding the earliest cases of epidemic disease are of supreme importance. "It is," Parkes announced, "universally and truly considered, that the inquiry into the origin of the first cases of an epidemic disease, in any locality, is a necessary preliminary to all other inquiries respecting the origin of future cases. At that period of the epidemic, the question is reduced into as simple elements as we can ever hope to find it in; and the influence of essential antecedents is less obscured than at a later date, by the presence of accidental and unnecessary circumstances."[12] Dealing only with Asiatic cholera, whose specificity provided an assured foundation for his inquiry, Parkes examined the origins of the great epidemic of 1848–1849.

As might be expected of a Board of Health associate, Parkes's special concern was in the etiological domain. He attacked the radical contagion-

---

11. Armand Trousseau, *Clinique médicale de l'Hôtel-Dieu*, 2 vols. (Paris: J. B. Baillière, 1861–1862), 1:175–176.

12. E. A. Parkes, "An Inquiry into the Bearing of the Earliest Cases of Cholera, which Occured in London during the Present Epidemic, on the Strict Theory of Contagion," *British and Foreign Medico-Chirurgical Review* 4 (1849): 251–276, passage cited, p. 251. See Pelling, *Cholera, Fever and English Medicine*, pp. 70–74.

ist view of cholera. His comments, however, have a broader bearing, for they address important aspects of epidemiological method.

> The first twenty-five or thirty cases [in an epidemic] are . . . most important. Did they arise together, or near each other? Were they exposed to contagion, from which the other inhabitants of the district were exempt? Can each successive case be traced to a prior case, until the patients are too numerous to be followed up? If these questions can be answered in the affirmative, it must be conceded that the strict contagionists have carried their point; if they are not so answered, then the observer has to seek for the cause of the early cases in other directions. It is necessary in examining evidence on this point to adopt two precautions. 1. Every reputed case of the disease must be known. 2. Every reputed case must be inquired into, and its exact nature determined; the loose accounts of bystanders and nonprofessional persons not being received as credible evidence.[13]

Parkes himself examined reports concerning more than thirty of the earliest cholera victims in London in the early autumn of 1848, paying particular attention to the possibility of personal contacts and thus of person-to-person transmission. He concluded that the causal agent of Asiatic cholera might in some cases have moved from person to person but that in numerous other cases no personal connection had occurred and causation was therefore to be assigned to changed local conditions. Each of the latter cases was an "independent manifestation" of the disease in a particular locality.[14]

Parkes thus ventured a mixed doctrine. In some cases, it seemed, contagion was real, but in other cases the occurrence of disease appeared to depend upon conditions independent of a contagious agent. Many of these cases had been examined by Parkes himself; others were described by medical men who were part of a concerted inquiry by the Board of Health into the circumstances surrounding the epidemic. The cases reported offered an apparently exhaustive record of the earliest days of the outbreak. What is notable here is not the conclusions reached, these being the familiar coin of Chadwick's legions, but the recognition that first cases were of central importance. Parkes's insistence upon and success in obtaining exact and complete information regarding these cases were equally significant.

He had pursued the exercise under seemingly most unfavorable circumstances. His domain was the world's greatest metropolis, a vast city with an ever-changing population and endlessly diverse economic activities and communications. Parkes's success in the detailed tracing of cholera cases

13. Parkes, "Inquiry into the Bearing of the Earliest Cases of Cholera," pp. 256–257.
14. Ibid., p. 274.

in a great city—a locale far removed from the often-stated ideal of a small rural epidemic situation—is explained by the unique and highly effective organization of London sanitary authorities during these severe cholera years. Here is a further lesson in the development of epidemiology and related public health matters, but one that cannot be developed here: confusions induced by scale can in fact be overcome, provided suitable administrative entities have been created and function according to plan. In the cholera epidemic of 1848–1849, the eager new Board of Health had insisted upon and obtained from physicians throughout London prompt reports of all confirmed and suspected cases of cholera that were encountered in practice. The circumstances of each case were then immediately investigated by the Board's own agents.

Timing thus favored Parkes's investigation, and the problem of localization appeared also to have been overcome. The results, however, remained ambiguous, principally because the conditions of the epidemic had not in fact been exhausted. Parkes realized this very well. The movement of Asiatic cholera across Europe revealed that many regions, by all outward signs favorable to the disease, had not been affected. Cholera, Parkes therefore proposed, was caused by a specific but unknown "poison." What also remained unknown, and this was the crucial epidemiological point, was the nature of an additional and clearly essential "element" that was "connected with the actual progress of the disease." When found, this missing element, and Parkes had no idea what it might be, would "complete the sum of conditions under which the poison attains its highest development."[15] Otherwise stated, the outbreak of individual cases of the disease indicated the necessary presence and action of a definite causal factor. What could not be explained, however, was why this factor, in conjunction with other requisite conditions, induced this or any other particular epidemic. Here Parkes set forward the epidemiological mystery of mysteries and clearly stated the issue that would soon provoke von Pettenkofer's ingenious *Bodentheorie*, the latter after 1860 becoming epidemiological orthodoxy in central Europe and also exercising a strong influence on certain physicians in Britain and India.

In epidemiology, on-site investigation greatly encourages accurate and more detailed coverage of events. Parkes literally cohabited London with epidemic cholera; he enjoyed, too, the services of a regular staff of medical investigators. His opportunity was also one of timing. A few years later, facing a different disease, Mélier and Buchanan also enjoyed this advantage of favorable timing. But now the circumstances were radically differ-

15. Ibid., pp. 273–274. Parkes offered as an acknowledged and unoriginal "conjecture" that an "atmospheric condition" peculiar to the autumn of 1848 may have been this element.

ent. Their field of operation was not a large metropolis but two remote port cities. On these occasions, however, distance no longer interposed its customary epidemiological difficulties.

Novel technologies dramatically assisted the study of epidemic yellow fever in Saint-Nazaire and Swansea. Mélier and Buchanan also benefited from improved administrative procedures. By the fourth decade of the nineteenth century both France and England had developed means for collecting and reporting to appropriate authorities numerous measures of the national condition, including such basic elements of vital statistics as the number of births, deaths, and marriages. In neither nation, nor in others where similar efforts were being made, was the collection of vital statistics complete or wholly reliable, and it was usually not prompt.[16] If, however, there were continuing and serious flaws in the routine operation of the new bureaucratic machinery, that same mechanism, built as it was upon a corps of interested regional and local authorities and working in close association with active medical practitioners, could respond quickly when an uncommon or serious threat arose. In 1828 Paris learned of the appearance of yellow fever in Gibraltar many weeks after the epidemic had begun. Thirty years later, she learned of yellow fever at Saint-Nazaire within a few days of its arrival; across the Channel, health authorities in London heard of the outbreak in Swansea no less quickly.

Epidemiology was being transformed by the mastery of time and space. Information gathered locally had always had to travel considerable distances to reach central authorities charged with general responsibility for protection of the nation from epidemic disease. In the 1840s these lines of communication were revolutionized by the widespread appearance of the railroad and telegraph. Post moving by rail traveled quickly and securely, and brief messages could be transmitted in minutes — messages such as the simple but decisive fact that a disease (i.e., yellow fever) had landed in a metropolitan port. Using the railroad, an experienced epidemiologist such as Mélier or Buchanan could and did reach an afflicted area within days, even hours, of the announcement of trouble, rather than within weeks or months. Epidemic diseases are diseases that move, often rapidly and widely, and successful study of their behavior demands that information and observers also move widely and with dispatch. The railroad and the telegraph assured such movement and thus constituted an important addition to the armaments of epidemiology. They created new epidemiological opportunities where before only the chance presence of a

16. There is no general history of the development of diverse national systems of vital registration, but the creation of the British system, a widely followed model for the coordination of collecting, marshalling and analyzing such data, has been admirably portrayed by Eyler, *Victorian Social Medicine*, pp. 37–65.

skilled observer had allowed careful circumscription of the early stages of an epidemic.

Atmospheric Theory and Epidemiology

Epidemiology is fated to play a social role. It is not simply that its subject, the human population, is a social object; rather, its conclusions bear directly on the social, economic, and political order and on the conduct of both public and private affairs. A generation ago, the historian of medicine Erwin H. Ackerknecht made this point particularly clear. Yellow fever, he pointed out in what has remained one of the most influential essays in the history of epidemiology, provoked most of the quarantine debates of the 1830s and 1840s. Yet quarantine was only the outward expression of deeper issues. In question were disease theory and consideration of the proper limits of state action. The central themes were, Ackerknecht argued, *"contagion and quarantines.* Quarantines meant, to the rapidly growing class of merchants and industrialists, a source of losses, a limitation to expansion, a weapon of bureaucratic control that it was no longer willing to tolerate, and this class was[,] quite naturally, with its press and deputies, its material, moral and political resources[,] behind those who showed that the scientific foundations of quarantine were naught. . . . Contagionism would, through its associations with the old bureaucratic powers, be suspect to all liberals, trying to reduce state interference to a minimum."[17]

More recently, Margaret Pelling has shown that this association cannot be so clearly drawn, especially because etiological positions were not in general sharply fixed.[18] The extreme noncontagionist outlook and radical contagionism were both minority viewpoints. In England, for example, the medical profession tended to take a cautious approach to etiology and to the epidemiological implications of etiology. Its position was essentially that of contingent contagionism. The base against which contingency was to be measured was noncontagionism, that is, no person-to-person transmission of disease. This base was in turn founded upon a further epidemiological proposition, namely, the causal role of the atmosphere in the communication of disease.

What was most striking and has subsequently proved most influential in Ackerknecht's argument was his identification of the social and economic

17. E. H. Ackerknecht, "Anticontagionism between 1821 and 1867," *Bulletin of the History of Medicine* 22 (1948): 587.

18. Pelling, *Cholera, Fever and English Medicine,* esp. pp. 295–310. Ackerknecht recognized that "contigent contagionism" was a common view; his purpose, however, was to exhibit the public role of noncontagionism (anticontagionism) and not to portray the full dimensions of the disputes of the period.

interests that were served by and that in turn propagated a particular theory of disease. Noncontagionism found especial favor among the manufacturing and commercial classes, for whom unrestricted communications were a necessary condition of mercantile and industrial expansion and prosperity. Freedom of movement, and economic freedom, were but other dimensions of personal liberty. Noncontagionism appealed also to a sizable body of reformers of various persuasions. To the classical liberal, noncontagionism was a welcome, additional argument to be used in his efforts to be rid of bureaucratic interference in economic and social life. It satisfied, too, his wish to break the tight hold of established parties and politicians on affairs of state.

Ackerknecht's argument loses much force if, as Pelling has shown, noncontagionism was a minority position. Yet, to still other observers, her criticism and revision of the Ackerknecht thesis seems insufficient. Ackerknecht exhibited the political dimension of the seemingly recondite matter of disease theory; Pelling has shown that the disease theory in question was not monolithic and that, in consequence, the medico-political connection must not be viewed as one of direct correspondence. But why, in fact, did this connection come into being in the first place? Why did disease theory so greatly concern practical men of affairs? That noncontagionism was congruent with liberalism is now accepted wisdom, even if the adherents to the two views were not always coextensive. But why and in what terms this congruence first came to be stated remains to be decided. Roger Cooter has suggested the domain in which an answer to these questions might best be sought.[19]

At issue is a matter of major significance not only for disease theory and criticism of quarantine but also for our principal concern, the articulation of epidemiological understanding and method. Cooter recalls Ackerknecht's emphasis on the activism inherent in the views of the noncontagionist party. He notes that this manipulative and domineering outlook characterized the values of the rising class of trade and industry, and he is aware that this interventionist attitude also characterized the Victorian sanitary party. Among the latter, the conviction reigned that relief in affairs of public health was to be found only through the sanitarian's mastery of water, filth, air, and other environmental factors affecting the human condition. Cooter connects this activism to an important consequence, namely, a wide-reaching effort to reconstitute the natural order of things. In the realm of medicine, this endeavor produced much more than a sim-

---

19. Roger Cooter, "Anticontagionism and History's Medical Record," in *The Problem of Medical Knowledge*, ed. P. Wright and A. Treacher (Edinburgh: Edinburgh University Press, 1983), pp. 87–108.

ple reclassification of diseases. It reflected, in Cooter's theory-laden words, a "process of reconstructing reality which was constitutive with the contemporaneous 'modernisation' of society, or process of increasing specialisation and fragmentation of the division of labour."[20] Cooter thus proposes to drive the analysis beyond the fact of a correspondence between formal (medical) knowledge and socioeconomic context (the claim advanced by Ackerknecht and modulated by Pelling) and to assay in detail how that correspondence was established and what social relations it reflected.

One need not wholly subscribe to Cooter's further contention that the noncontagionist position was in reality a program designed to wrest control of the conditions of existence from the people, or even accept the calmer proposition that it revealed the imperative of science working against the people or counter to the common understanding, to appreciate his suggestive comments regarding the role assigned by disease theorists to atmospheric influence.[21] As has been noted repeatedly throughout this volume, the notion of atmospheric influence was the central proposition of noncontagionist doctrine; medical environmentalism, especially when faced with the problem of communicable disease, traditionally found in air its most effective agency. The sociopolitical role of this influence was equally important, for the predominance of the atmosphere meant the diminution of other, potentially influential, relations. It served, Cooter suggests, to diminish those activities by which individuals discern and develop mutual interests and to degrade the medical, especially epidemiological, meaning of interpersonal relations.

This in turn suggests a decidedly lesser role for, and interest in, the possibility of person-to-person communication of disease; that is, atmospheric predominance renders impotent the contagionist argument. To assert the priority of atmospheric disease causation thus served to maximize the influence of factors beyond the control and probably beyond the comprehension of ordinary persons. The atmosphere imposed social and epidemiological distance and seemed to assure the impotence of the common or prudent man in such matters. The way was thus opened to the specialist. Cooter concludes: "Air, once the very stuff of human breath, became in this body of thought an alien 'thing' amenable only to the analytical understandings and moral and political interventions of environmental manipulators."[22]

So it would seem, yet even the specialist had no easy task in attempting to comprehend and, especially, dominate the atmosphere. Atmospheric

20. Ibid., p. 98.
21. Ibid.
22. Ibid., p. 99.

causation of communicable disease offered a manifold of interpretive possibilities; the atmosphere as cause or as the vehicle for the transmission
of a causal agent seemed prepared to provide virtually any needed solution. Here, unhappily, was and is the problem: the atmosphere lent itself
poorly to exact study. The first evidence of its maleficent condition seemed
usually to be the smells that it conveyed. A foul or putrid odor might well
presage or accompany the appearance of a dread disease. This odor was
not the spontaneous product of the atmosphere itself. It usually reflected
the fact that the air had taken up an emanation that had arisen from decay-
ing organic matter or perhaps simply from unspecified filth. This emanation might be gaseous or it might be composed of extremely fine particles.
In either case, the emanation seemed, save for the odor that betrayed its
presence, beyond human apprehension and in itself subject to no further
scientific or epidemiological analysis.

Concern for the influence of the atmosphere had been an intrinsic element in classical medical doctrine, notably in the Hippocratic treatise *Airs,
Waters and Places,* as well as in a large number of subsequent hygienic
texts. It later played a major role in the efforts of the seventeenth-century
English clinician, Thomas Sydenham, to create a new basis for the classification of diseases. Following the botanical model, Sydenham identified
fixed disease species but was compelled also to account for the many variations that were observed, particularly variations in the epidemic behavior
of communicable diseases. He determined that seasonal and longer-term
changes were present, and that these changes in the character, frequency,
and intensity of epidemics were produced most directly by changes in the
atmosphere (the so-called annual and epidemic constitutions). Sydenham's
influence was immediate and long-lasting and contributed greatly to the
prosperity of the atmospheric doctrine during the eighteenth century, now
comfortably established as a comprehensive and relatively consistent secu-
lar explanation of the coming and going of epidemic disease. When fears
of pestilential disease became newly acute towards 1800, the notion of an
etiologically active or disease-inducing atmosphere stood ready to aid interpretation and to guide preventive measures.[23]

The seeming advantage of the atmosphere as the basic element in epidemiological explanation was that it provided a multifaceted explanation
of otherwise inexplicable events. But again, its great disadvantage was its

23. On these large themes, see Genevieve Miller, "Airs, Waters and Places in History,"
Journal of the History of Medicine 17 (1962): 129–140; J. C. Riley, "The Medicine of the
Environment in Eighteenth-Century Germany," *Clio medica* 18 (1983): 167–178; L. J. Jor-
danova, "Earth Science and Environmental Medicine: The Synthesis of the Late Enlighten-
ment," in *Images of the Earth: Essays in the History of the Environmental Sciences,* ed.
L. J. Jordanova and R. S. Porter (n.p.: British Society for the History of Science, 1979), pp.

inherent unspecificity. The atmosphere assured social distance, no doubt, but it possessed too many possibilities to be used alone as a rigorous instrument for the assessment of an epidemic or as grounds for explaining that epidemic. Virtually all parties in Gibraltar had invoked atmospheric causation, and virtually all had found it satisfactory. They did so, however, for various and inconsistent reasons. It seemed that there was no way that the atmosphere could be manipulated, conceptually or physically. Even self-styled specialists found no way to create a widely acceptable ground for understanding disease transmission or to serve as a well-articulated basis for agreed-upon disagreement. The condition of the atmosphere could be described verbally and certain of its features expressed in numbers, yet neither exercise offered sufficient grounds for rigorous determination of the origin or movement of an epidemic disease. The perception of the supposedly critical factor, smell, varied wildly with the observer.

To become epidemiologically meaningful, these several variables not only had to be determined with precision but compared systematically and consistently with other factors such as geographical location, disease incidence, and mortality. Presumably, too, comparisons would need to be made with other epidemic outbreaks. Comparisons of this kind were a mainstay of early epidemiological reasoning, yet therein lay the problem. The degree of correlation between one or another "cause" — say atmospheric temperature or humidity (to offer only measurable quantities) — and a given "effect" — for example, the incidence of yellow fever in Gibraltar or Saint-Nazaire — could be inferred only in qualitative and usually highly subjective manner, if at all. When a chain of causes was brought into question, the situation only worsened. The ensuing multiple effects simply could not be resolved into a set of mutually dependent links, links each of which was well characterized and whose interrelationships and collective effect were precisely specified. Despite these problems, atmospheric influence did continue to provide the most frequent explanation of those epidemics that struck many persons suddenly and within a relatively restricted area.

119–146; C.-E. A. Winslow, *The Conquest of Epidemic Disease* (Princeton: Princeton University Press, 1943; reprint, Madison: University of Wisconsin Press, 1980), pp. 161–175; Major Greenwood, "Sydenham as an Epidemiologist," *Proceedings of the Royal Society of Medicine*, Section on Epidemiology and State Medicine, 12 (1918–1919): 56–76; Owsei Temkin, "An Historical Analysis of the Concept of Infection," in *The Double Face of Janus and Other Essays in the History of Medicine* (Baltimore: Johns Hopkins University Press, 1977), pp. 456–471. Margaret Pelling's discussion (*Cholera, Fever and English Medicine*, passim) is essential. On the fate of environmental factors in the bacteriological era, see Johanna Bleker, "Die historische Pathologie, Nosologie und Epidemiologie im 19. Jahrhundert," *Medizinhistorisches Journal* 19 (1984): 33–52, esp. pp. 48–49 and her references; the school of Max von Pettenkofer long continued to resist the exclusivist claims of medical bacteriology.

But it served this function only in the face of abundant counterinstances and by leaving much unexplained. What atmospheric explanation gained by its assertion of the general reasons for the outbreak of an epidemic, it lost in the detailed assessment of the course of that epidemic. In fact, it offered little or no guidance to persons who wished to explore these details. As we have seen, however, it was just this matter of detail that played the crucial role in attempts to place epidemiology on secure scientific foundations.

The atmospheric theory enjoyed high favor in the early nineteenth century; no doubt it did so in part because of its agreement with emerging liberal political values. But that favor and this connection provided unsure foundations for the creation of epidemiology, despite the obvious fact that this science assumed form and won public recognition within the then-leading liberal societies, France and England. If, as Cooter has maintained, the special virtue of atmospheric causation to the liberal apologist was that it provided a scientific explanation that derived from and insisted upon social distance (a view which propounded the cognitive priority of an "external depersonalized environment") the historian should not halt his inquiry with this, the liberal's credo or conclusion.[24] One must attempt to determine precisely how, in the minds of accepting physicians and publicists, this maleficent atmosphere was understood to act.

To some, Chervin and his many followers being the foremost examples, atmospheric influence, in conjunction with unsanitary local conditions contributory to that influence, seemed to act according to the broader or dual formula of medical doctrine and political conviction. To others, however, the political motif was either softly spoken or altogether absent. Unless we care to stress self-unawareness or even dissimulation, neither Mélier nor Buchanan nor even Simon, himself a prominent public figure, made much of the socioeconomic rationale associated with noncontagionism. To these students of communicable disease, the atmosphere constituted only one albeit important element in the constellation of conditions and causes surrounding an epidemic. They treated their science in increasingly phenomenological manner. It is hard to imagine how, in their case, an ideological stance of maintaining "social distance," even within the terms of one's scientific theory, can be squared with the research that underlay that theory, namely, case-tracing within the context of specific time and place and possible personal contacts.

Obviously, as part of the needed unpacking of the objective and ideological components of early epidemiological inquiry, it is essential to consider independently the two elements of the old equation, noncontagion

24. Cooter, "Anticontagionism and History's Medical Record," p. 98.

and nonimportation of disease (that is, abandonment of quarantine). The new open-mindedness of the epidemiologist in the field, and such we have met at work in the 1860s, arose from a willingness to reconsider the legitimacy of this supposedly intimate union. In the course of this reconsideration there emerged the possibility of a far more flexible approach to the problem of controlling the introduction of epidemic disease. Cooter's assessment and conclusions may thus fit well the earlier years of the yellow-fever debates, the era of Chervin and his critics, but they are not suited to the later period, that of the 1860s as illustrated by the investigations conducted in Saint-Nazaire and Swansea. What had changed was the physician's method of inquiry and his new sense of the efficacy in the domain of popular persuasion of the (seemingly) neutral conclusions of science. He had learned, too, a lesson of capital importance to all epidemiological inquiry, namely, the epidemiological distinctiveness of communicable diseases, this to be added to clinical circumscription and, wherever possible, etiological specificity, of each such disease. He also knew that, in such difficult matters as those pertaining to the spread of a deadly disease, methods had now been devised and were being intelligently applied that proved adequate to the task of capturing fundamental features of the crucial matter, the movement of the disease.

Whatever, then, its ideological burden, the workaday task of epidemiology was recognized to be to trace the movement of a disease or diseases through a discrete population. Behind the epidemiologist's quest lay the sick individual. But the latter belonged primarily to the practicing physician; the epidemiologist took the community as his responsibility. From his analysis of the conditions that favored or discouraged the movement of disease, he could attempt to derive measures that might counteract the further spread of the epidemic or prevent the outbreak of another. More sanguine observers also believed that such analyses might provide clues to the specific cause of disease and epidemic. But in the 1860s there was general agreement that first must come the study of local social and environmental conditions, and these should be treated in as exhaustive and exact a manner as possible. Here is met early epidemiology in the doing and here, too, are met inquirers such as Mélier and Buchanan.

The investigations of the yellow-fever epidemics at Saint-Nazaire and Swansea were descriptive and relatively complete. Buchanan, and especially Mélier, verged on offering a veritable ecology of the disease. These inquiries required that a given epidemic situation be explored in depth and throughout its duration. It was possible to meet these needs because of the singular appropriateness of the two localities and the timing of each inquiry. "In depth" meant not simply a willingness to examine all potentially relevant factors (some of which were found, soon enough, to be irrelevant), but the desire to do so in a systematic, reasoned manner, which itself was a function not only of expectation and previous experience but of the phenomena that were encountered in the course of the inquiry.

Mélier's work, and that of Buchanan four years later, drew little attention to the traditionally prominent matter of etiology. Rival disease theories, they seemed to say, should follow and not lead epidemiological investigation. In the 1860s frustration with conventional etiological explanations, whether noncontagion or contagion, had reached a peak. A fresh alternative, the germ theory of disease, had only just begun to assume form and receive experimental confirmation; it was destined later to conquer the epidemiological field. Early epidemiology, however, made its stand on the use of case-tracing and the scrupulous assessment of local environmental conditions. The fundamental phenomenon was disease transmission, and the basic problem was to discover the modalities of this transmission. Neither case-tracing nor assessment of local conditions was new, yet, when pursued with system and care, they provided a comprehensive and reliable portrait of epidemic yellow fever such as had not previously been available. From this portrait could be read important scientific and practical lessons: yellow fever is in fact an imported disease, whatever be its cause, and the disease can be controlled in nonendemic areas by vigorous sanitary intervention in ports maintaining communications with tropical lands. The response to yellow fever at Saint-Nazaire became an example for others to follow, and many did. But the creation of the portrait deserves equal emphasis, for the study of yellow fever at Saint-Nazaire and Swansea provided a second model, one of epidemiological method.

Bibliographical Note
Index

Bibliographical Note

THE PRINCIPAL SOURCES upon which this book is based are *Documens recueillis par MM. Chervin, Louis et Trousseau, membres de la commission française envoyée à Gibraltar pour observer l'épidémie de 1828; et par M. le Dr. Barry, médecin des armées anglaises*, 2 vols. (Paris: Imprimerie royale, 1830); François Mélier, "Relation de la fièvre jaune survenue à Saint-Nazaire en 1861," *Mémoires de l'Académie impériale de médecine* 26 (1863): 1–223, also "Discussion" by several voices of this work in *Bulletin de l'Académie impériale de la médecine* 28 (1862–1863): 646–695, 834–891, 977–1039 [Mélier's report plus the discussion were also published together as a separate volume in 1863]; "Report by Dr. George Buchanan on the Outbreak of Yellow Fever at Swansea," *Parliamentary Papers* 33 (1866) [Reports from Commissioners. 17. Pollution of Rivers. Public Health; i.e., Eighth Report of the Medical Officer of the Privy Council, with Appendices, 1865], pp. 440–468, also John Simon, "III. Foreign Epidemics of the Year and the General Question of Contagion in its Bearings on the Public Health. 3. Yellow Fever at Swansea," ibid., pp. 30–46.

On the eventful history of yellow fever, see H. R. Carter, *Yellow Fever. An Epidemiological and Historical Study of Its Place of Origin* (Baltimore: Williams and Wilkins, 1931); H. H. Scott, *A History of Tropical Medicine*, 2 vols. (Baltimore: Williams and Wilkins, 1939), 1:279–453; and L. J. B. Bérenger-Féraud, *Traité théorique et clinique de la fièvre jaune* (Paris: Octave Doin, 1890); also W. G. Downs, "The Story of Yellow Fever since Walter Reed," *Bulletin of the New York Academy of Medicine* 44 (1968): 721–727. The character of the disease is fully portrayed in G. K. Strode, ed., *Yellow Fever* (New York: McGraw-Hill, 1951), and more recent developments are presented by W. G. Downs, "History of Epidemiological Aspects of Yellow Fever," *Yale Journal of Biology and Medicine* 55 (1982): 179–185. Important contemporary accounts of the disease are René La Roche, *Yellow Fever, Considered in its Historical, Pathological, Etiological, and Therapeutical Relations*, 2 vols. (Philadelphia: Blanchard and Lea, 1855); Wilhelm Griesinger, *Infectionskrankheiten, Malariakrankheiten, gelbes Fieber, Typhus, Pest, Cholera* [Rudolf Virchow, ed., *Handbuch der speciellen Pathologie und Therapie*, Bd. II, 2ᵗᵉ Abteilung] (Erlangen: F. Enke, 1857), pp. 59–86; expanded discussion in the second edition of 1864.

The fundamental study of the socioeconomic and political context of the early European yellow-fever epidemics is G. D. Sussman, "From Yellow Fever to Cholera. A Study of French Government Policy, Medical Professionalism, and Popular Movements in the Epidemic Crises of the Restoration and the July Monarchy" (New Haven: Ph.D. diss., Yale University, 1971); see also the influential essay by E. H. Ackerknecht, "Anticontagionism between 1821 and 1867," *Bulletin of the History of Medicine* 22 (1948): 562–593. British epidemiological thought at midcentury is thoroughly analyzed by Margaret Pelling, *Cholera, Fever and English Medicine, 1825–1865* (Oxford: Oxford University Press, 1978); also the several essays in *Times, Places, and Persons. Aspects of the History of Epidemiology*, ed. A. M. Lilienfeld (Baltimore: Johns Hopkins University Press, 1980). The broader medical setting and the focus of French hygienic thought are depicted in E. H. Ackerknecht, *Medicine at the Paris Hospital, 1794–1848* (Baltimore: Johns Hopkins Press, 1967); A. F. La Berge, "The Early Nineteenth-Century French Public Health Movement: The Disciplinary Development and Institutionalization of *hygiène publique*," *Bulletin of the History of Medicine* 58 (1984): 363–379; William Coleman, *Death Is a Social Disease. Public Health and Political Economy in Early Industrial France* (Madison: University of Wisconsin Press, 1982).

Two articles dealing directly with the subject of this book are William Coleman, "Epidemiological Method in the 1860s: Yellow Fever at Saint-Nazaire," *Bulletin of the History of Medicine* 58 (1984): 145–163, and C. E. Gordon Smith and M. E. Gibson, "Yellow Fever in South Wales, 1865," *Medical History* 30 (1986): 322–340.

Questions of quarantine are discussed by Léon Colin, "Quarantines," *Dictionnaire encyclopédique des sciences médicales*, 100 vols. (Paris: Victor Masson, P. Asselin, 1869–1889), 80:3–171; J. C. McDonald, "The History of Quarantine in Britain during the 19th Century," *Bulletin of the History of Medicine* 25 (1951): 22–44; Norman Howard-Jones, *The Scientific Background of the International Sanitary Conferences* (Geneva: World Health Organization, 1975).

Index

DESIGNED BY BRUCE GORE
COMPOSED BY METRICOMP, GRUNDY CENTER, IOWA
MANUFACTURED BY BOOKCRAFTERS, CHELSEA, MICHIGAN
TEXT AND DISPLAY LINES ARE SET IN PALATINO

Library of Congress Cataloging-in-Publication Data
Coleman, William, 1934–
Yellow fever in the North.
(Wisconsin publications in the history of science
and medicine: no. 6)
Bibliography: pp. 197–198.
Includes index.
1. Epidemiology—History—19th century. 2. Yellow
fever—France—Saint-Nazaire—Epidemiology—History—
19th century.   3. Yellow fever—Wales—Swansea (West
Glamorgan)—Epidemiology—History—19th century.
4. Yellow fever—Gibraltar—Epidemiology—History—
19th century. I. Title. II. Series. [DNLM:
1. Epidemiologic Methods. 2. History of Medicine,
19th Cent.—Europe. 3. Yellow Fever—history—Europe.
W1 WI805 no. 6 / WC 532 C692y]
RA649.C64 1987   614.4'09   86-40456
ISBN 0-299-11110-5
ISBN 0-299-11114-8 (pbk.)